Shawn's Self-Care Routine:
A Boy's Guide to Healthy Habits

Danielle M. Jackson

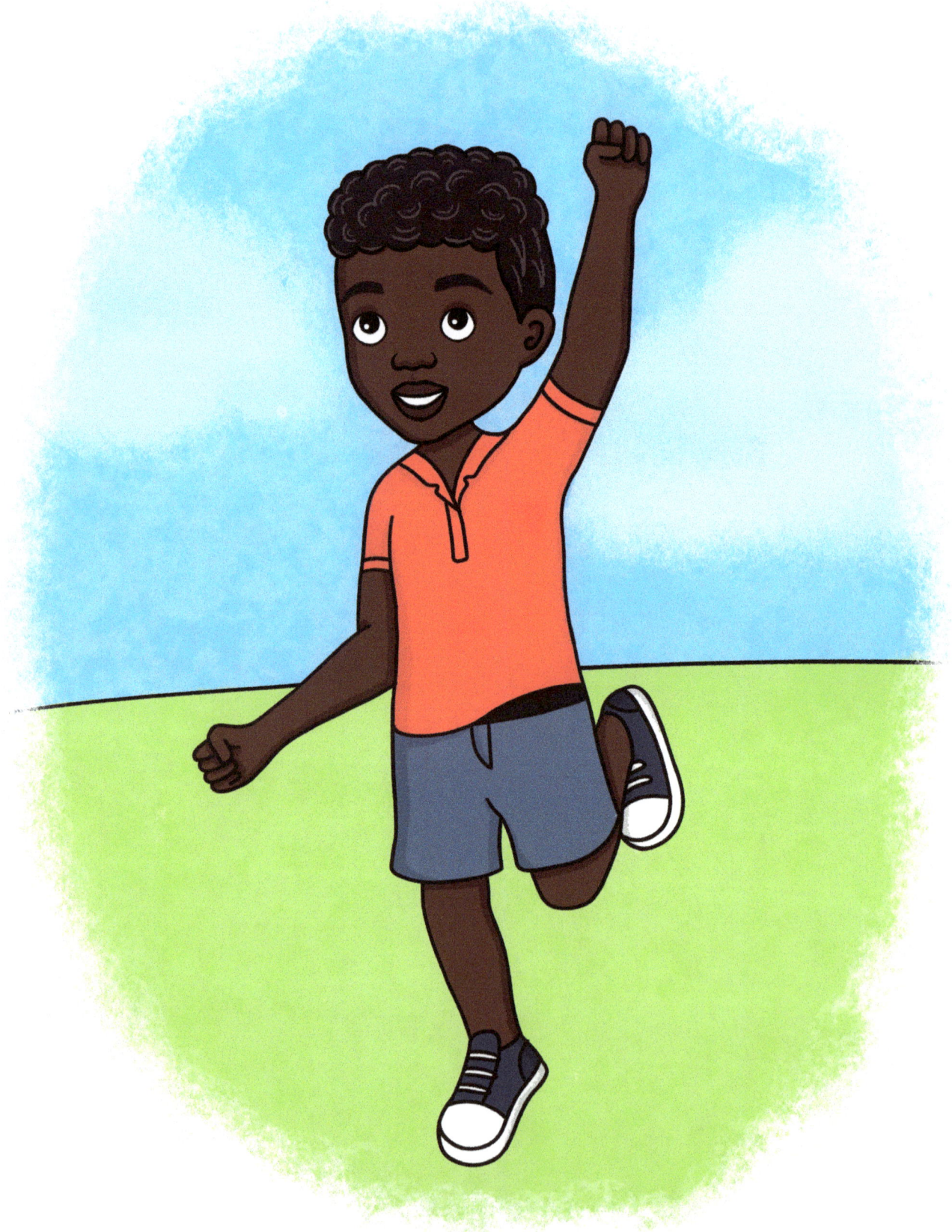

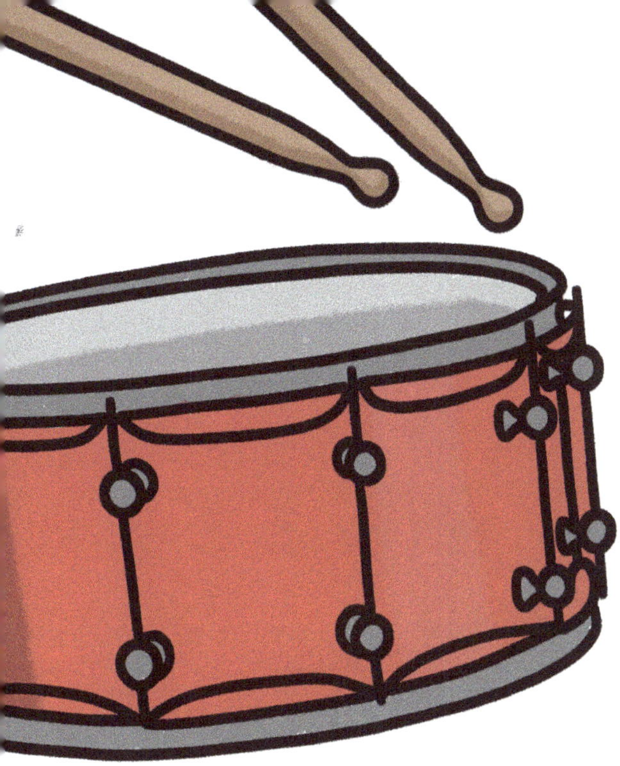

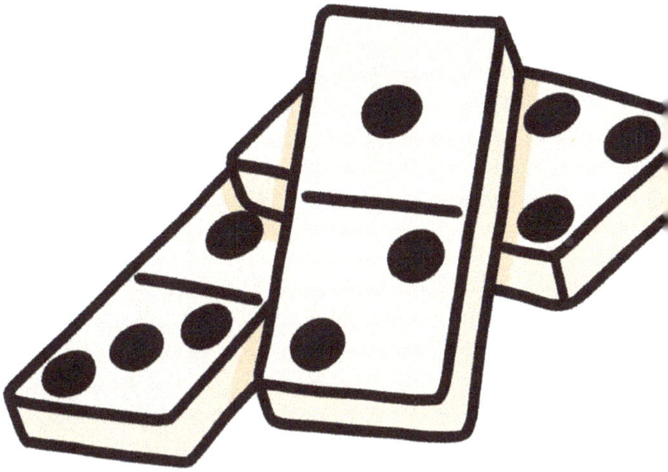

Shawn enjoys his self-care routine. He established this routine because school-life balance allows him to be his best self.

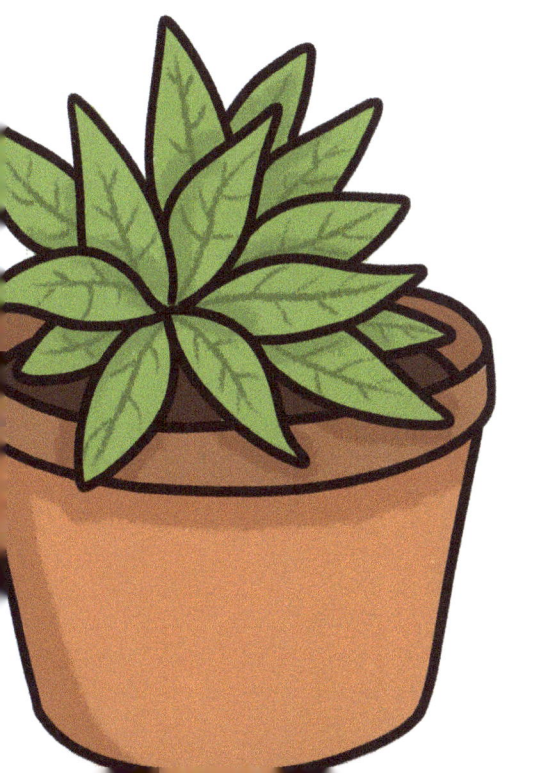
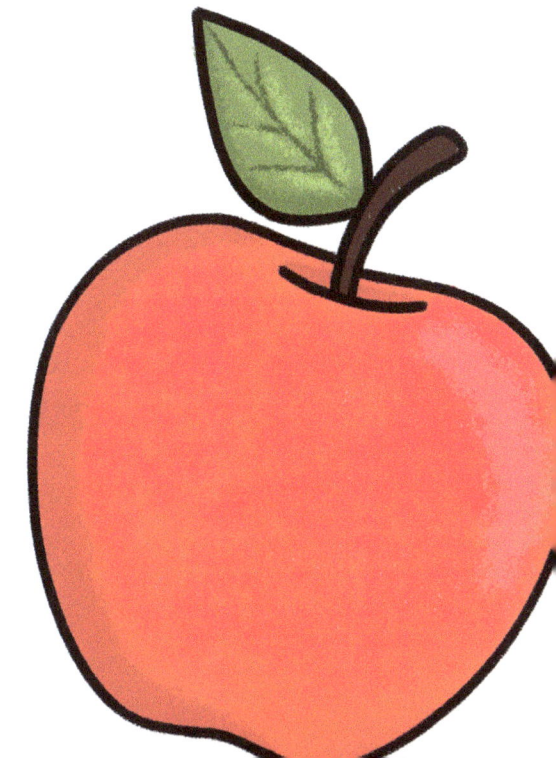

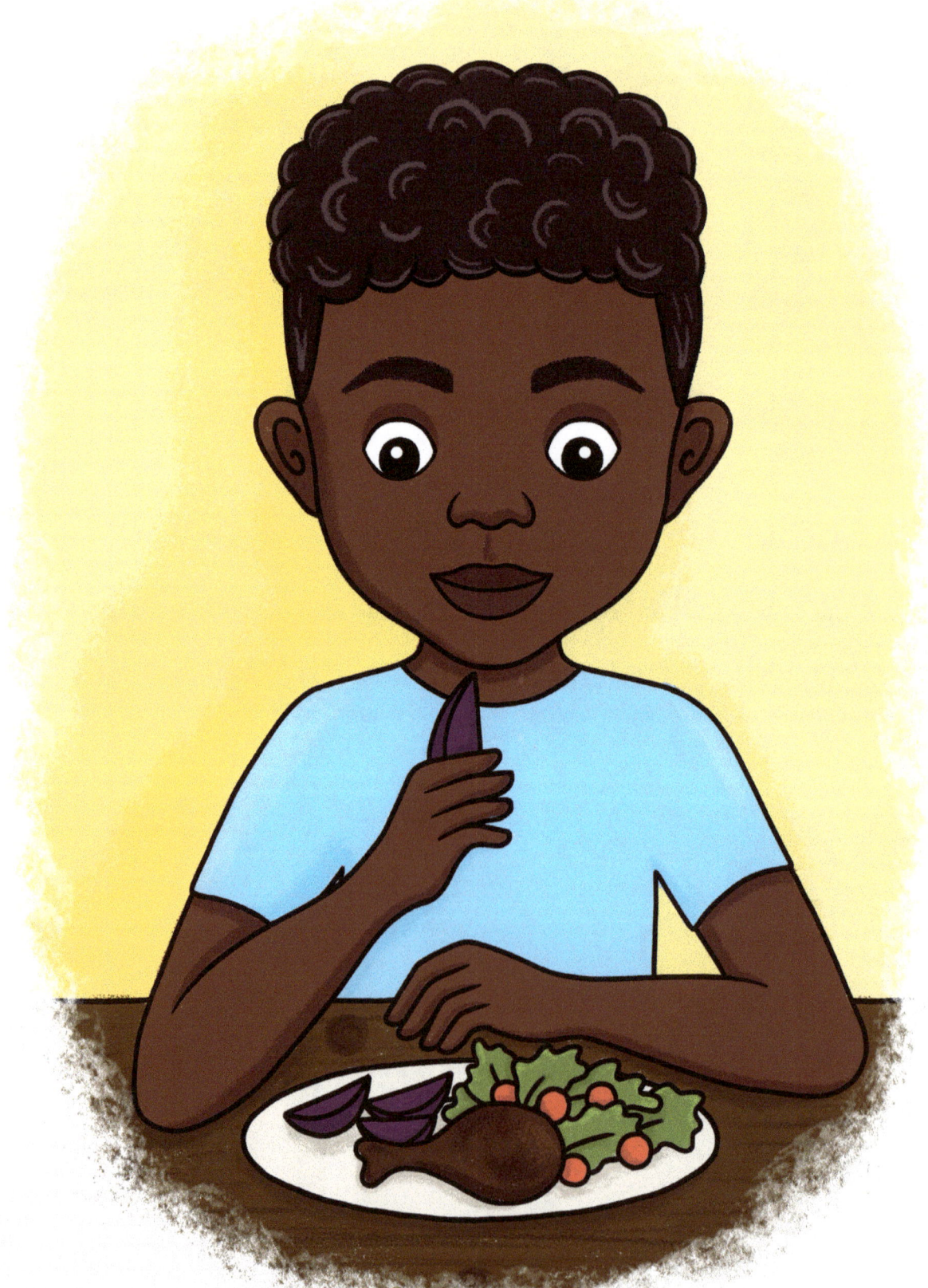

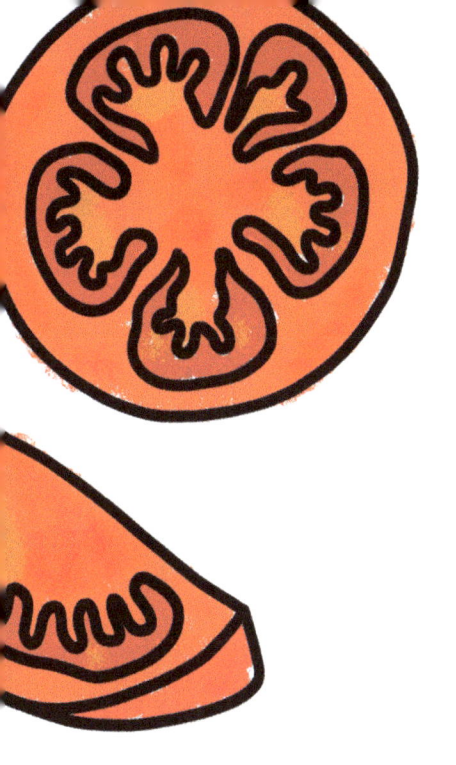
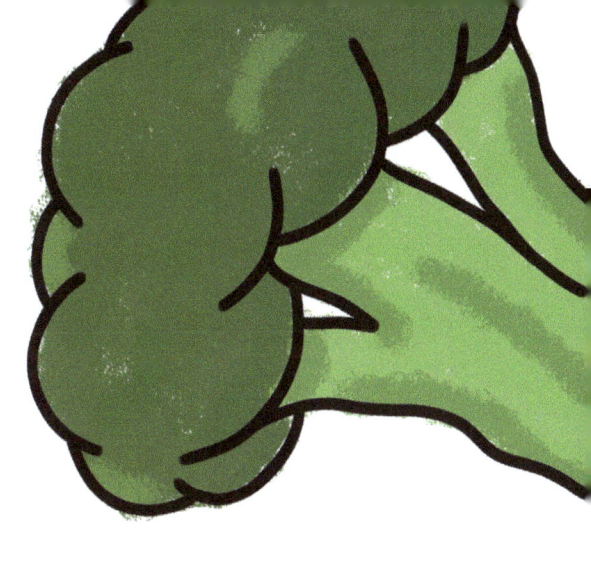

Shawn makes it his business to eat foods that help his body perform well. He appreciates foods that are not only nutritious but delicious.

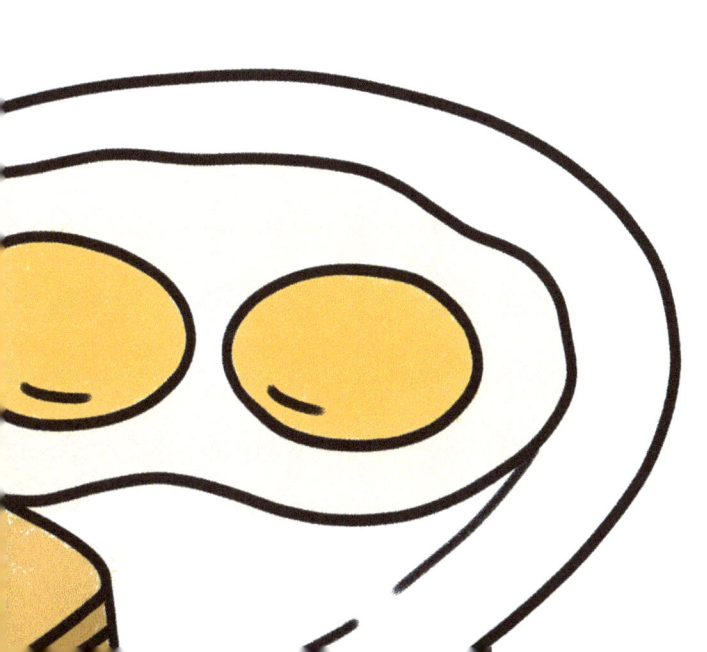
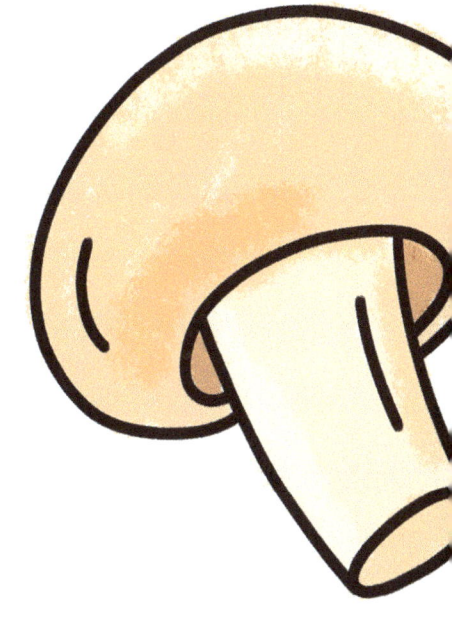

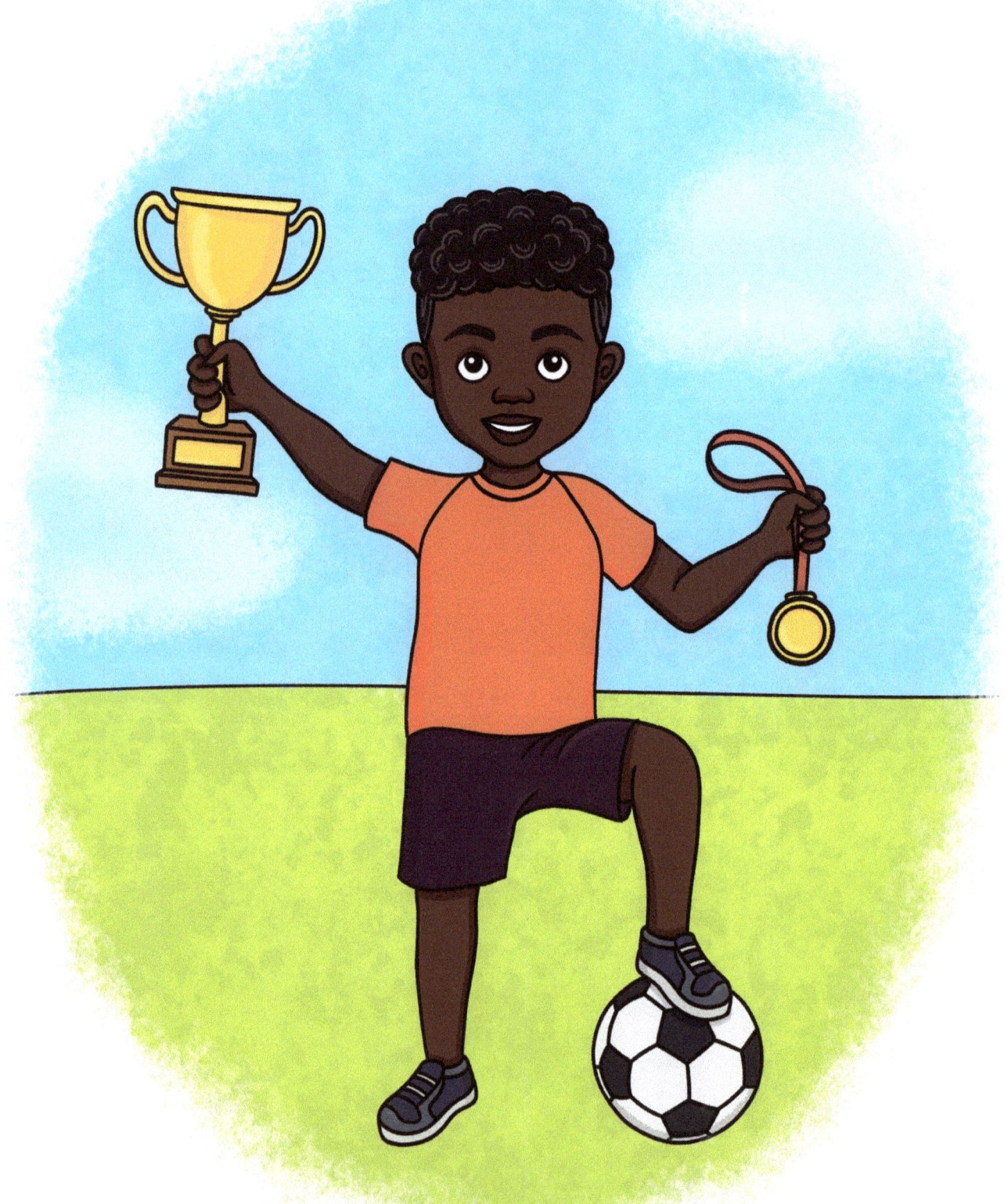

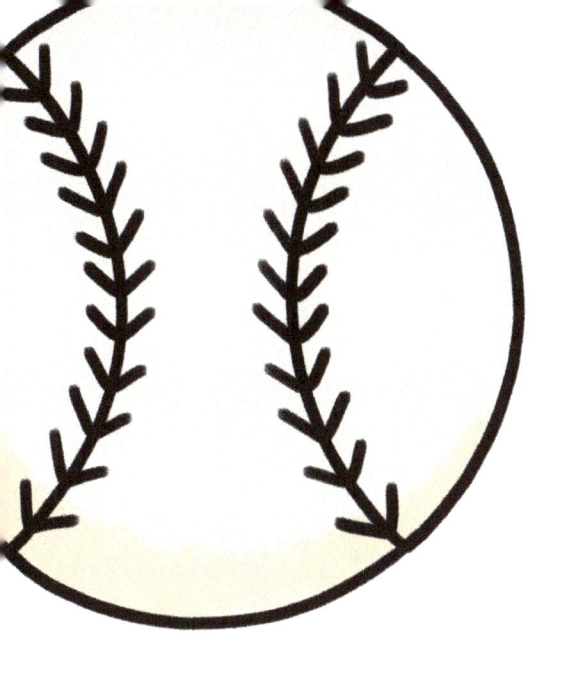
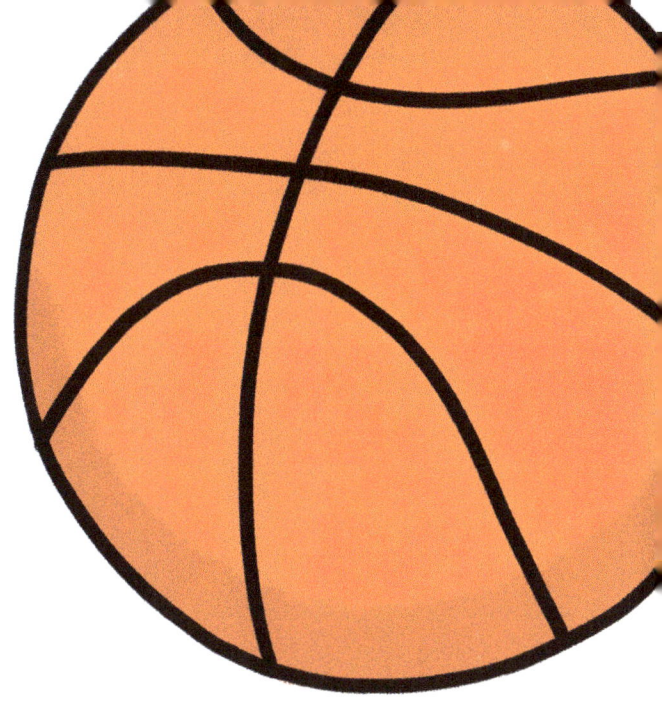

Staying active by playing sports allows Shawn to keep his body strong. Sports also teach him good sportsmanship skills, helping him become a leader on and off the field.

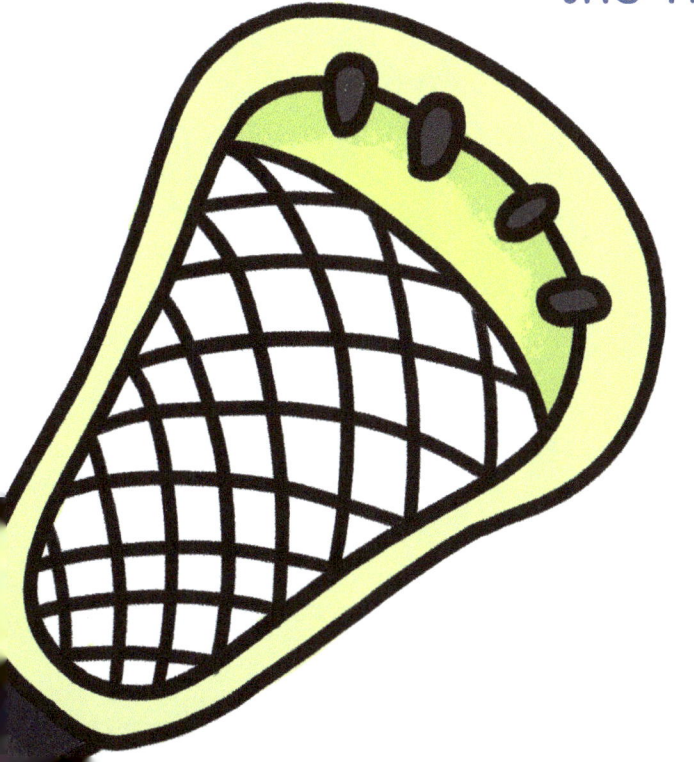
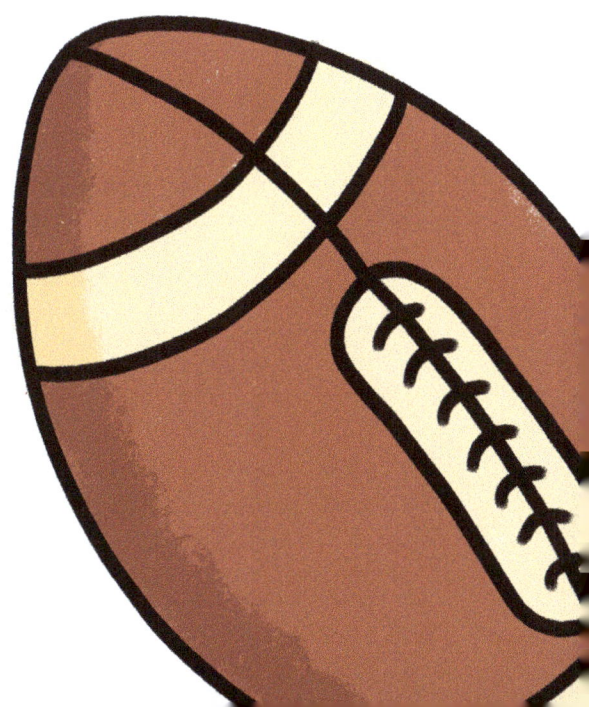

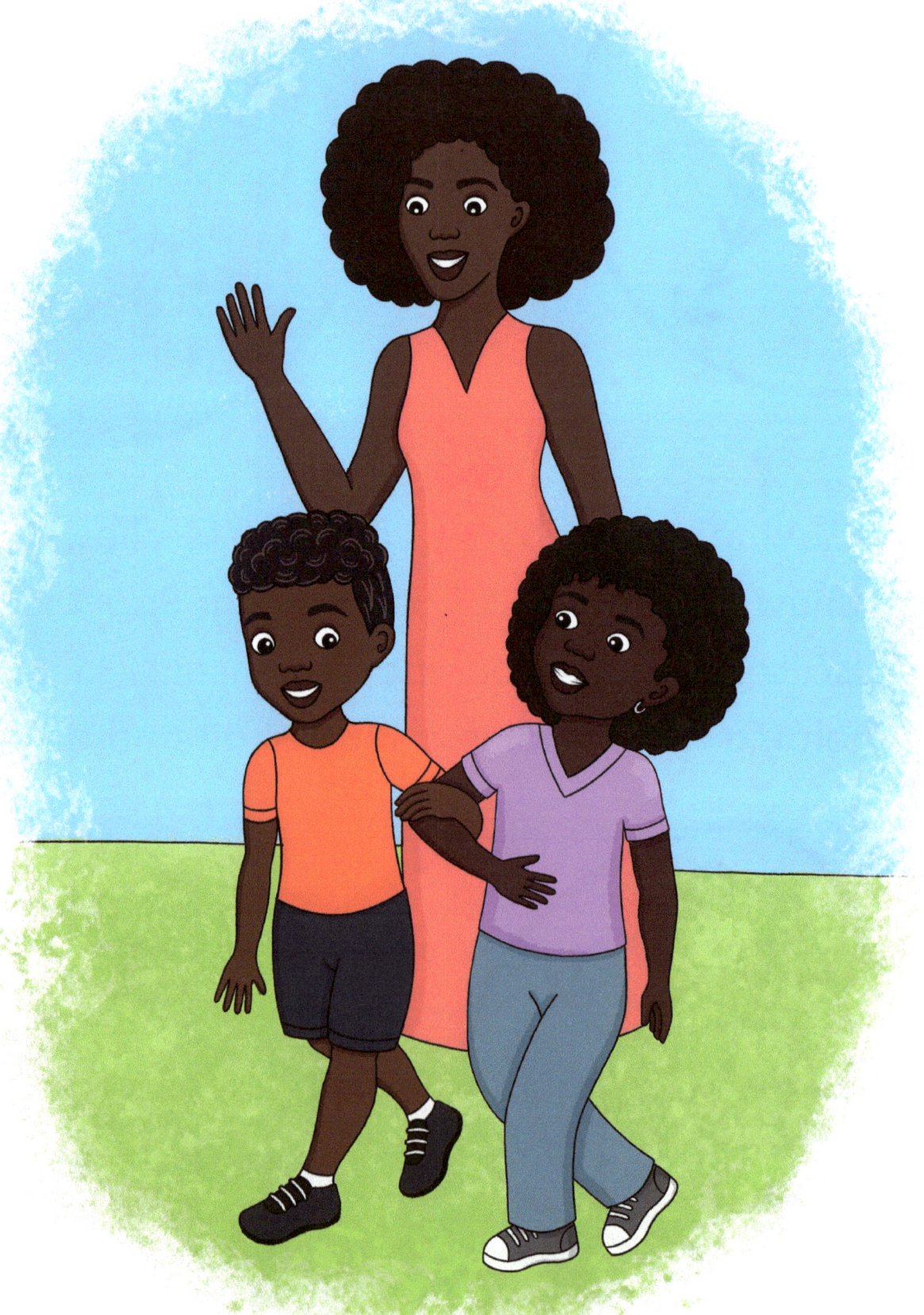

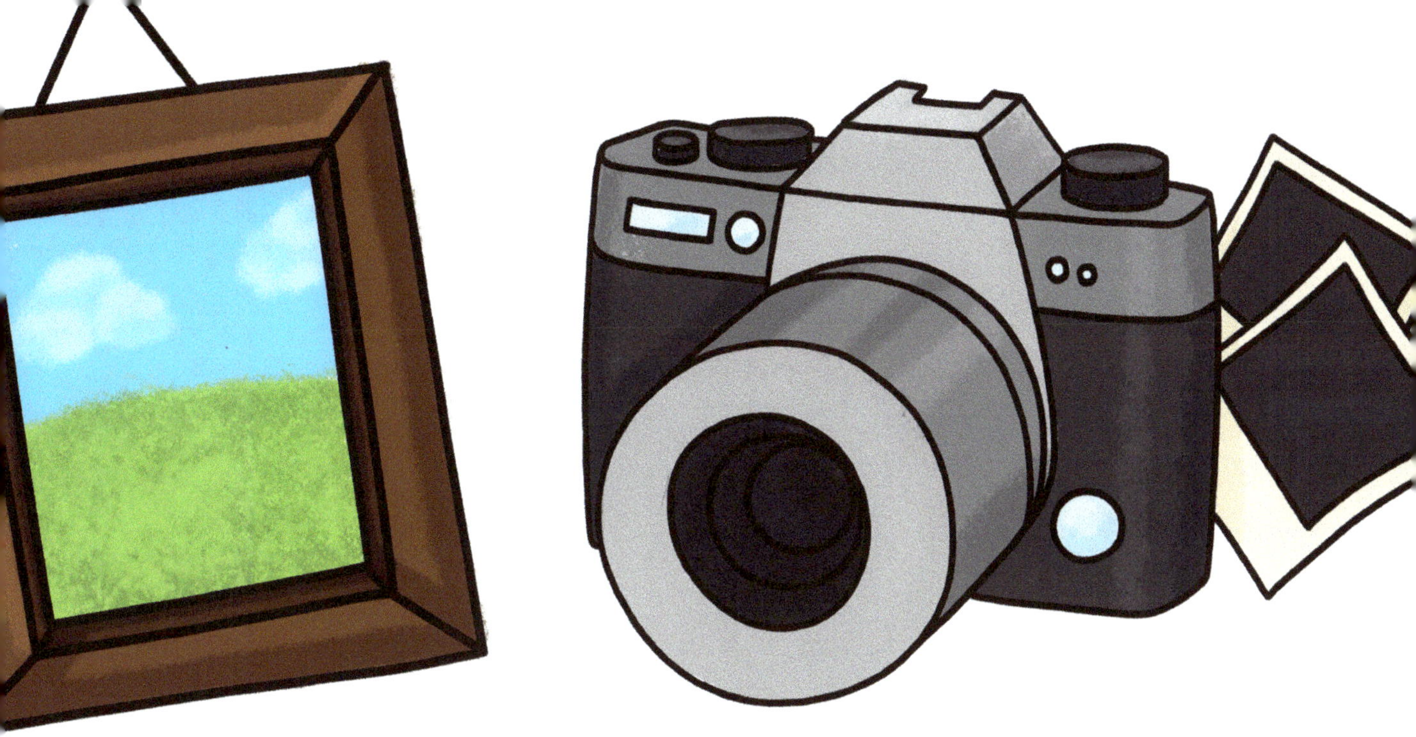

Let the good times begin! Shawn adores his family and friends along with the beautiful memories they create together.

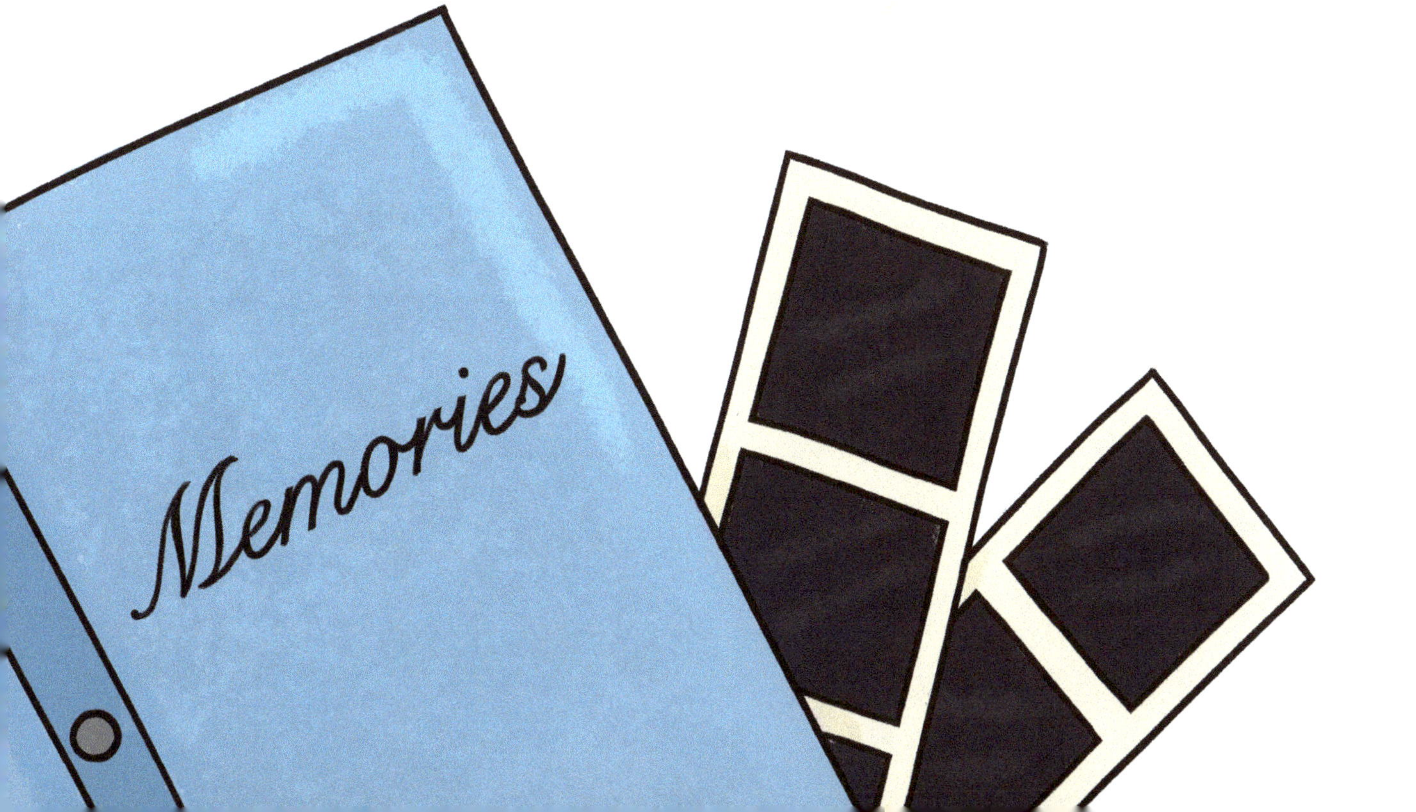

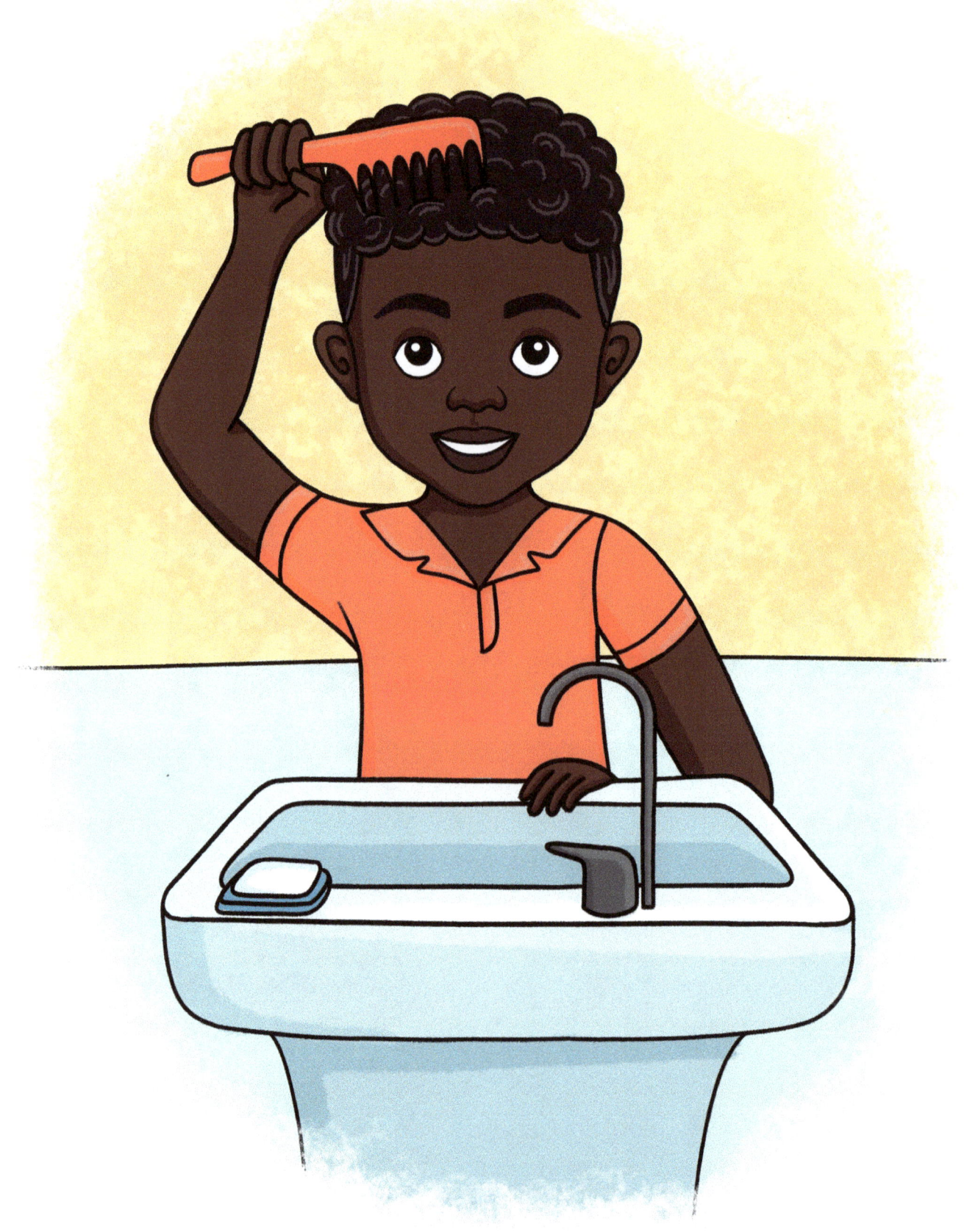

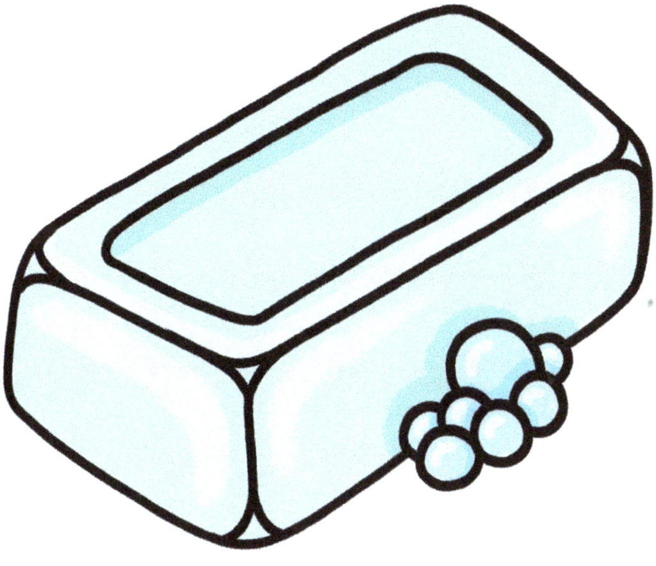

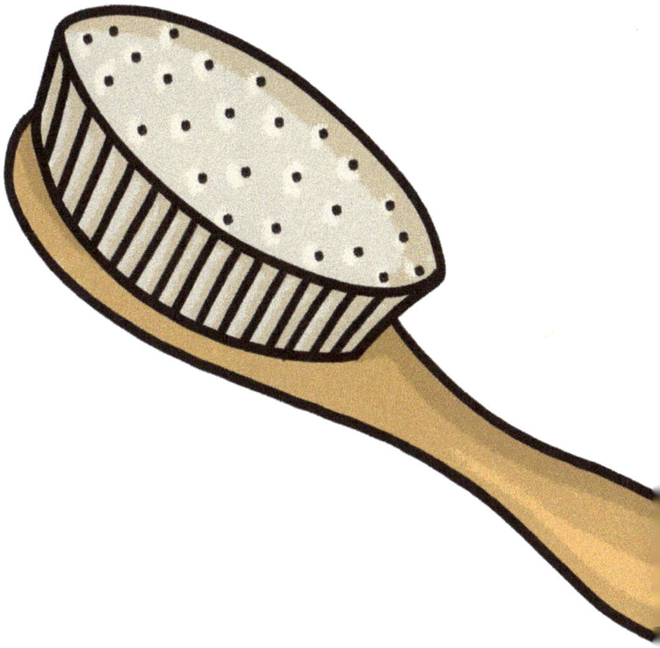

Grooming allows Shawn to present the best version of himself every day.
He knows that if you look good, you'll feel good.

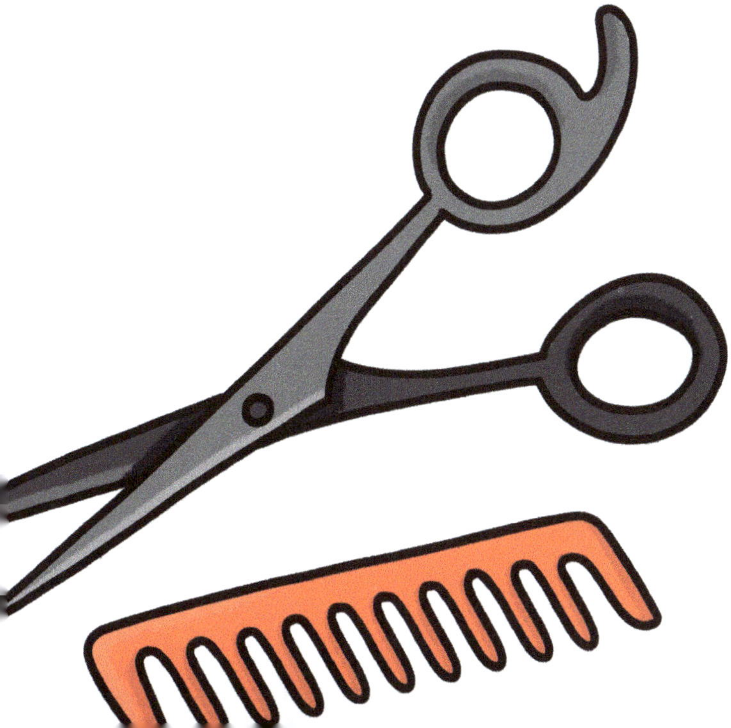

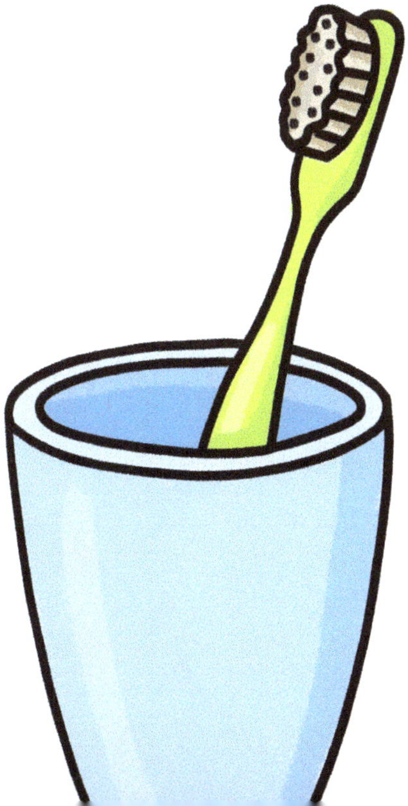

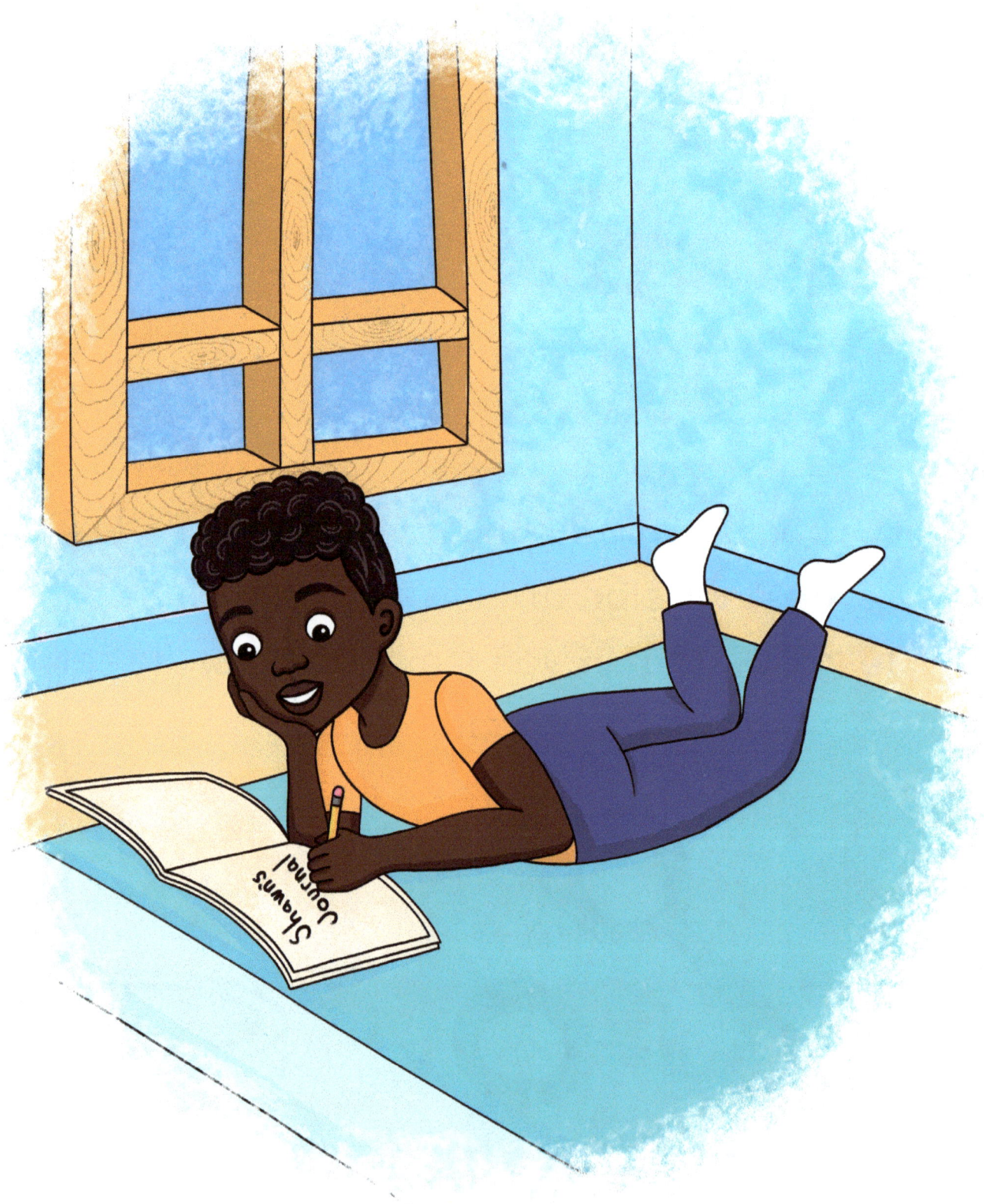

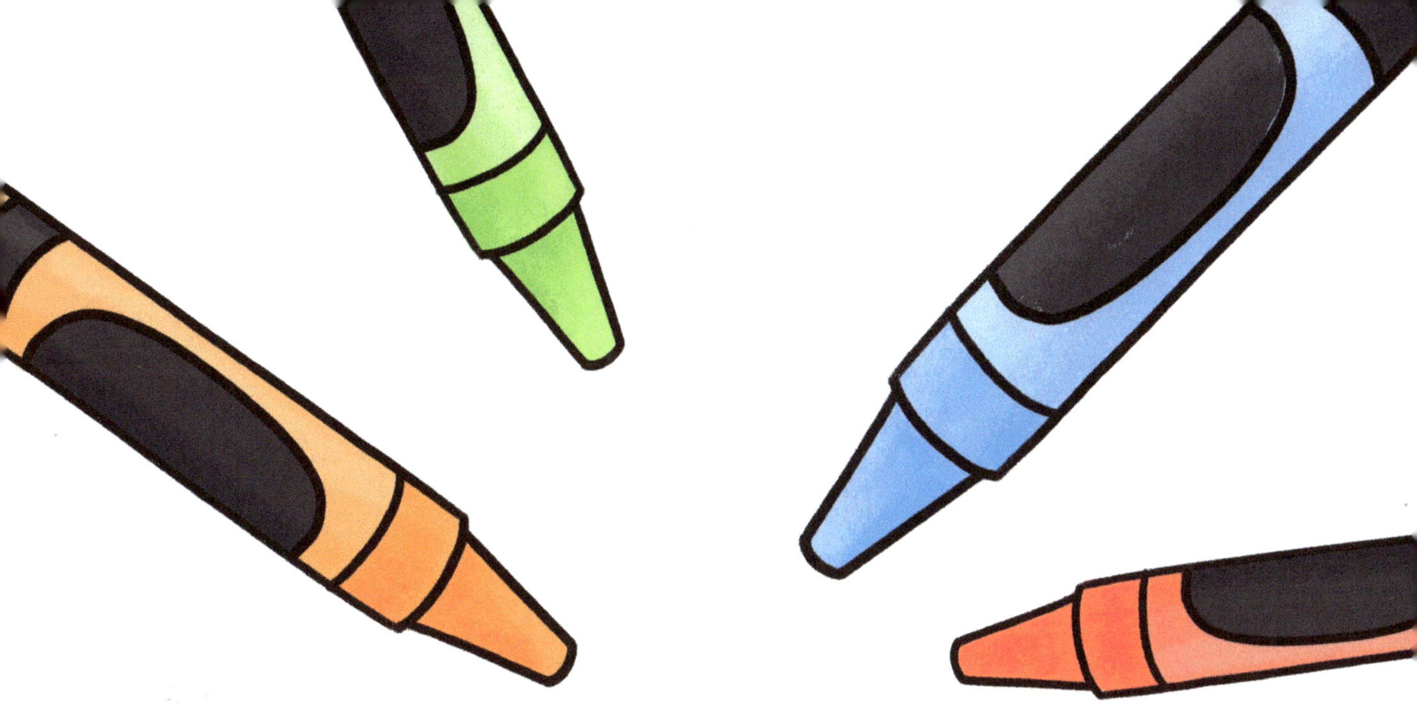

Journaling is Shawn's way of organizing and processing his personal thoughts. By keeping a journal, he is free to express his emotions privately.

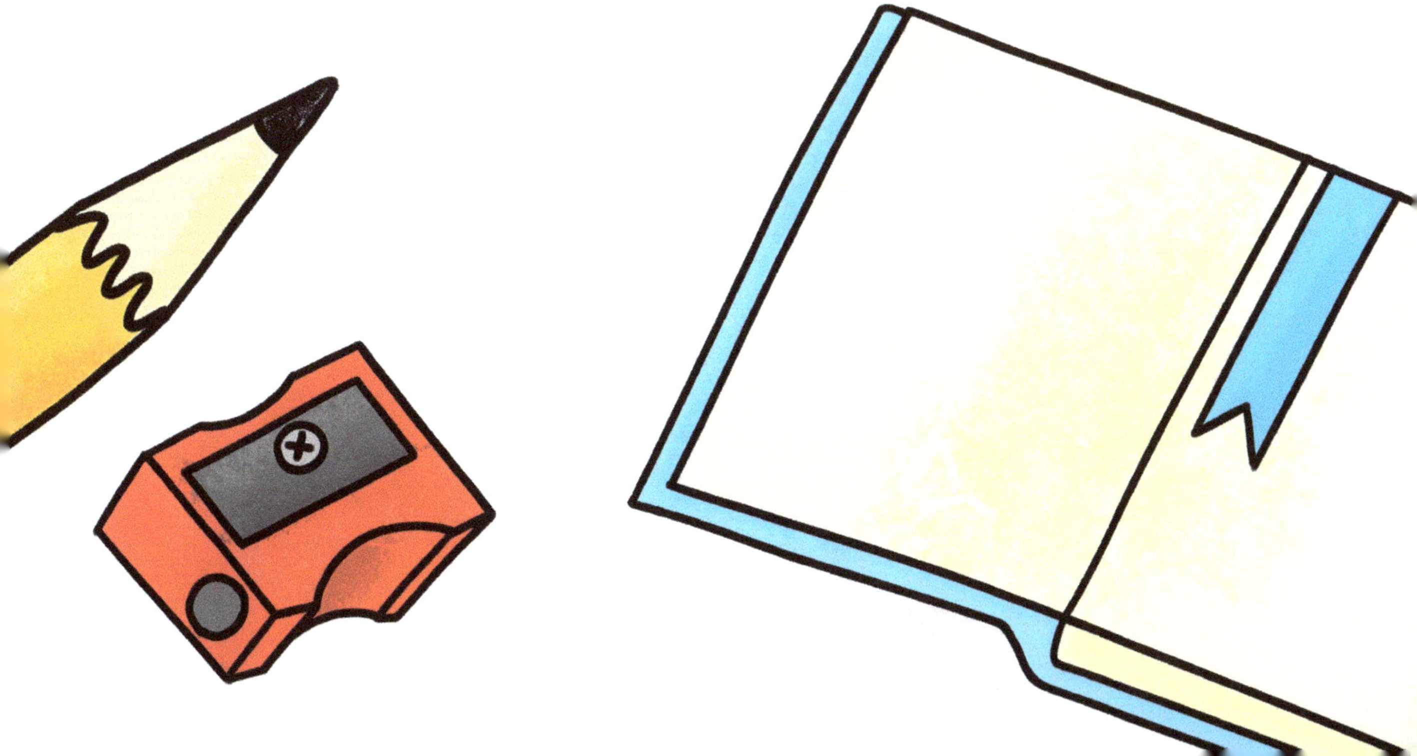

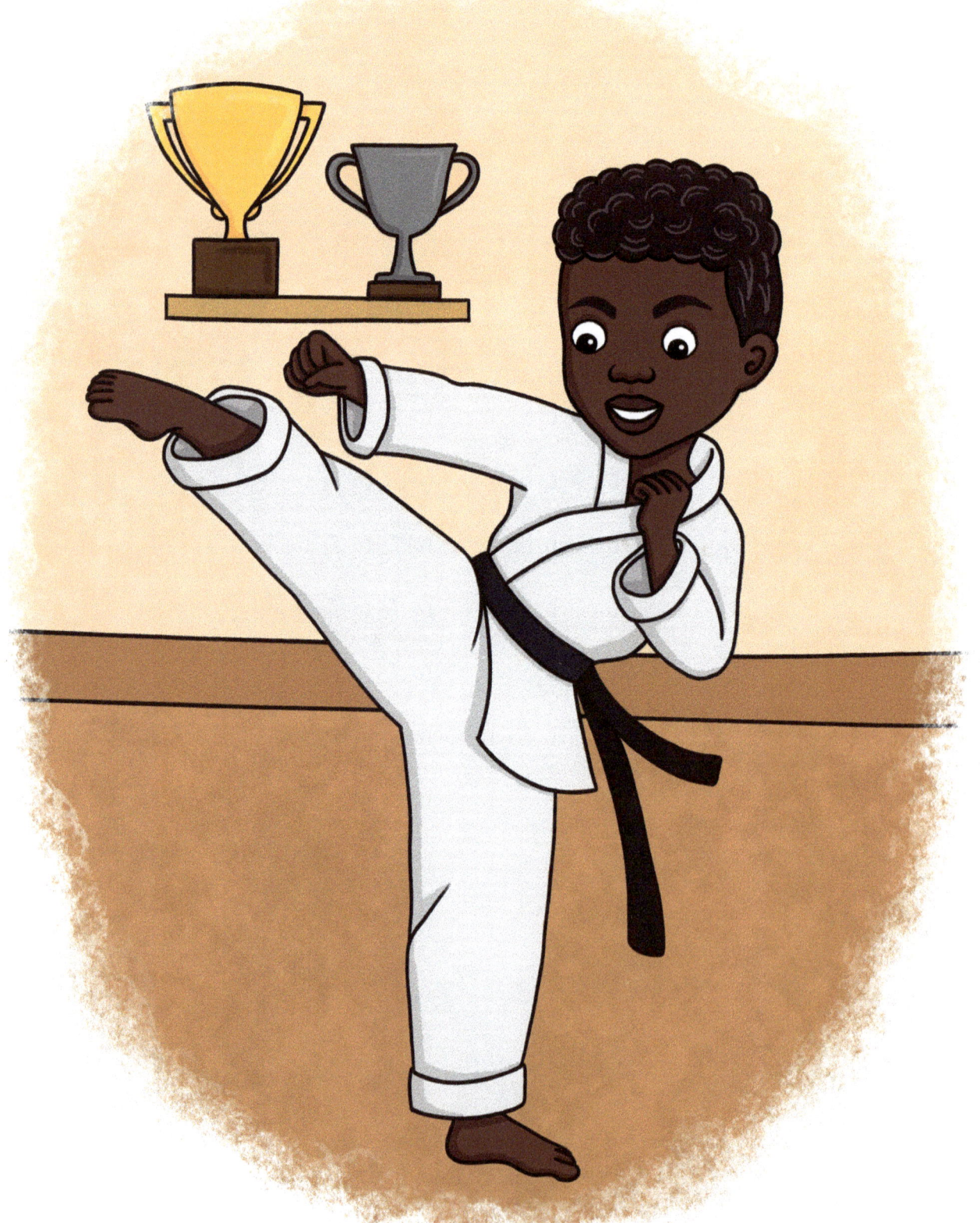

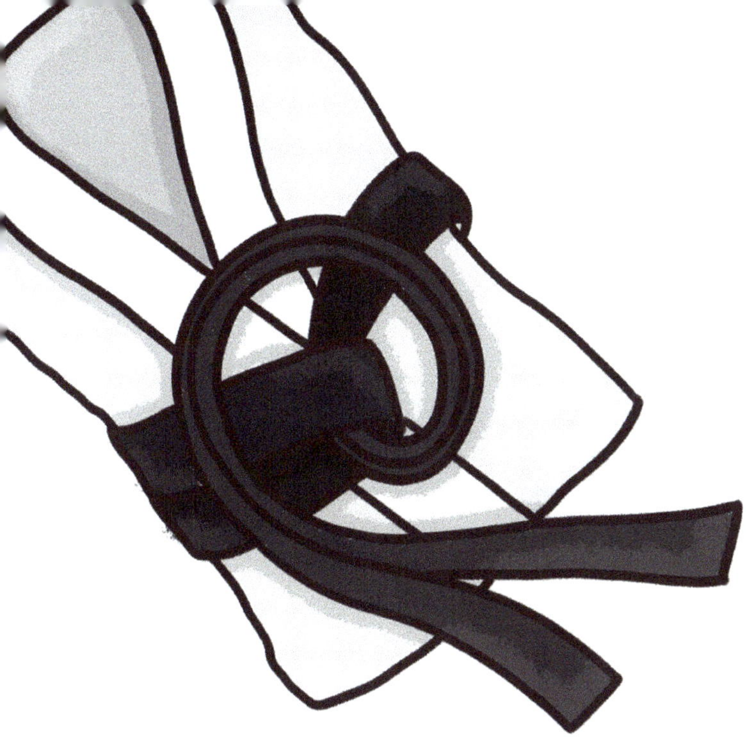

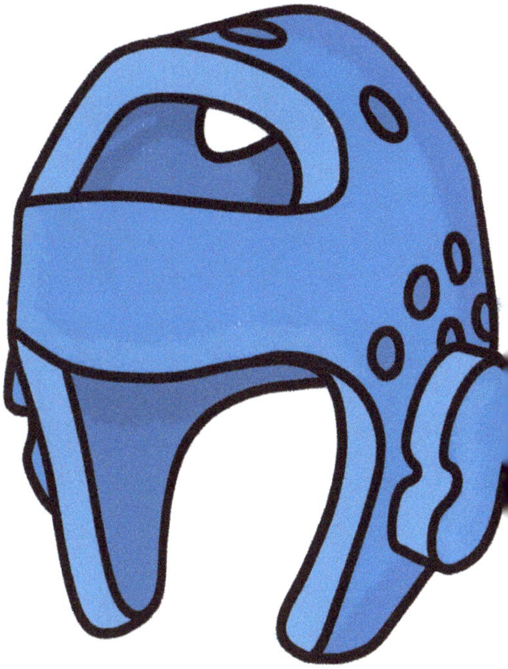

Shawn's ability to master techniques in martial arts helps him develop his character. He takes pride in learning a skill that challenges him to grow while working towards achieving a black belt.

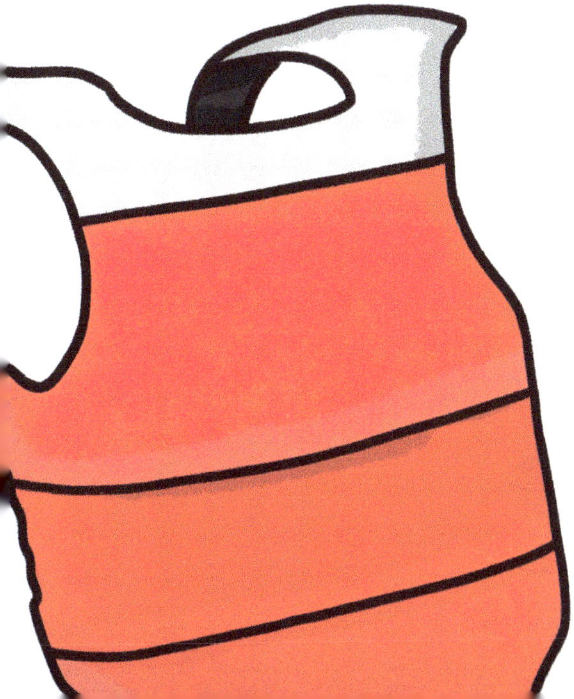

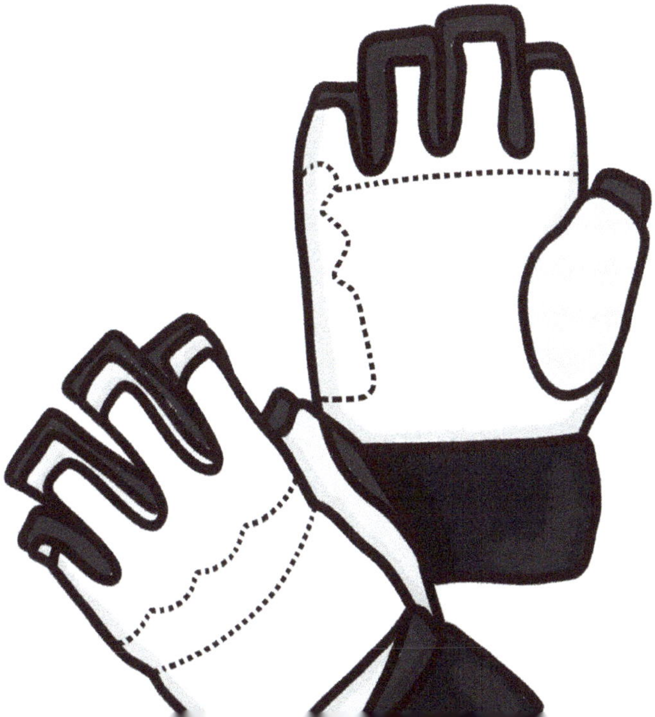

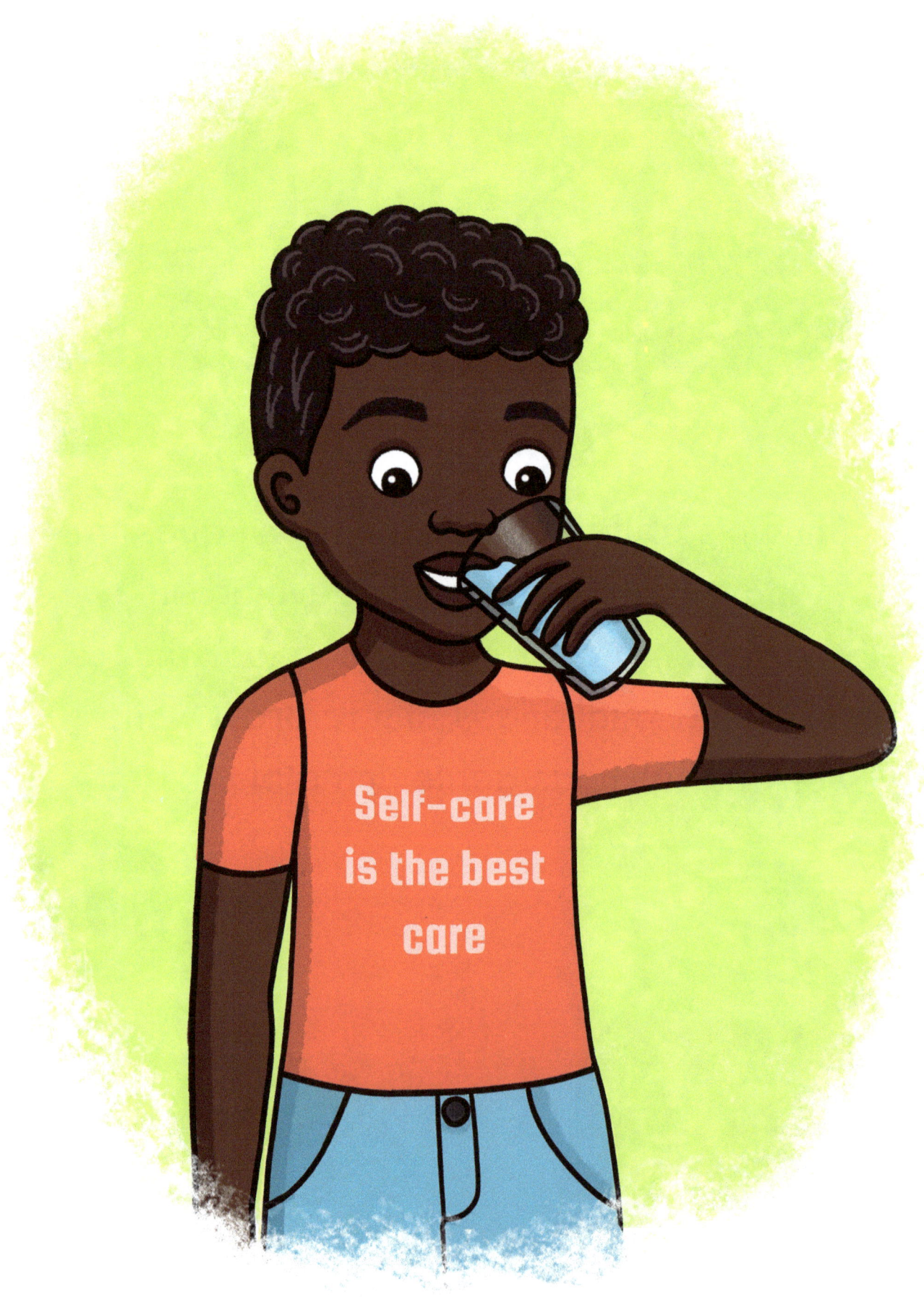

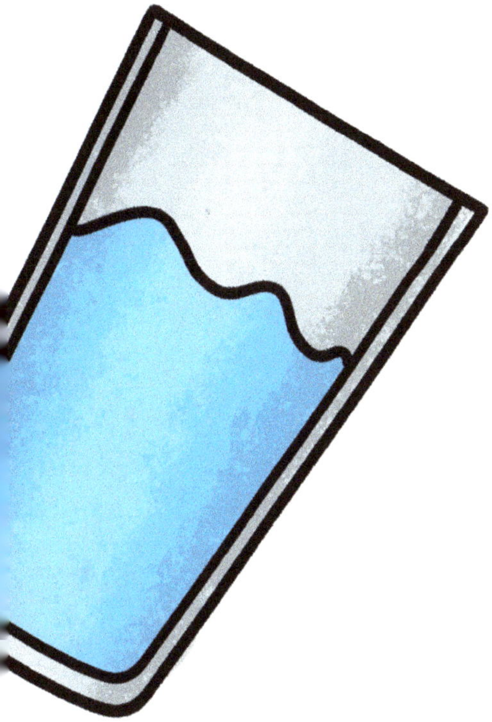

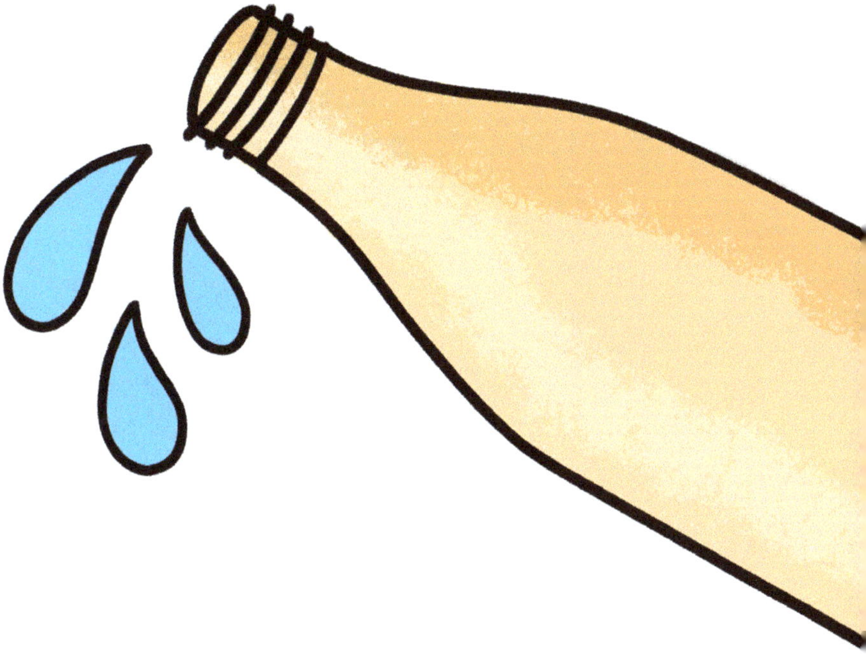

Water is just what the body ordered. Shawn enjoys drinking his fair share of water to quench his thirst and help his body stay hydrated and healthy.

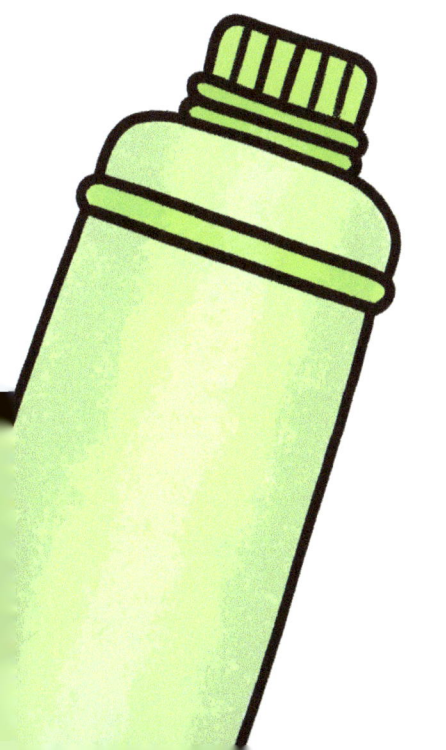
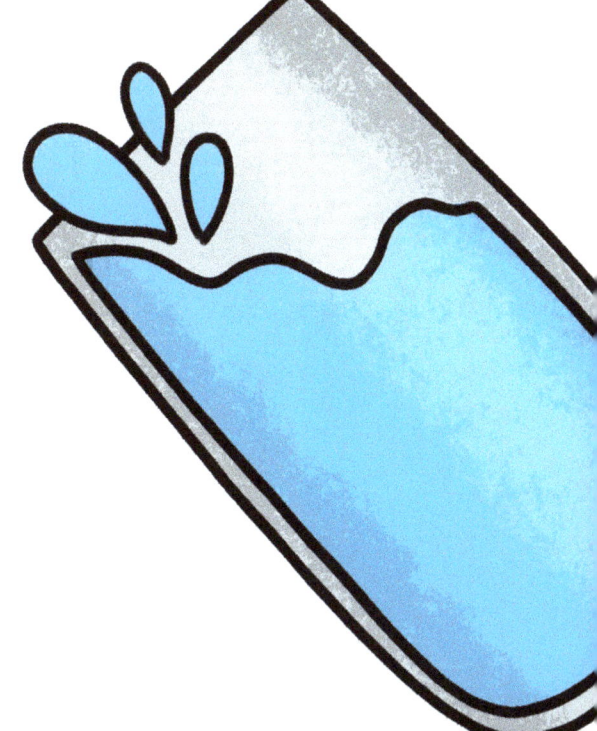

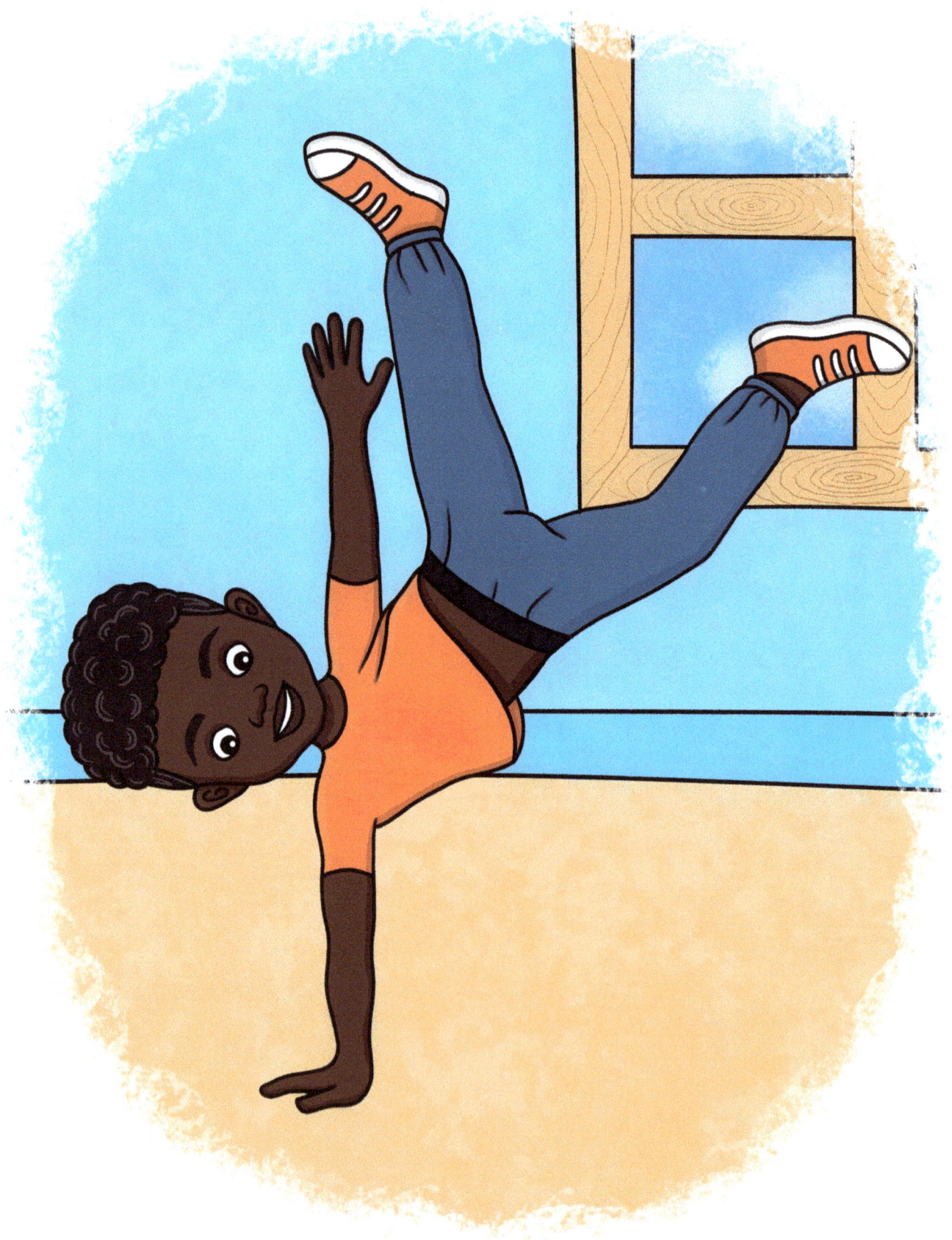

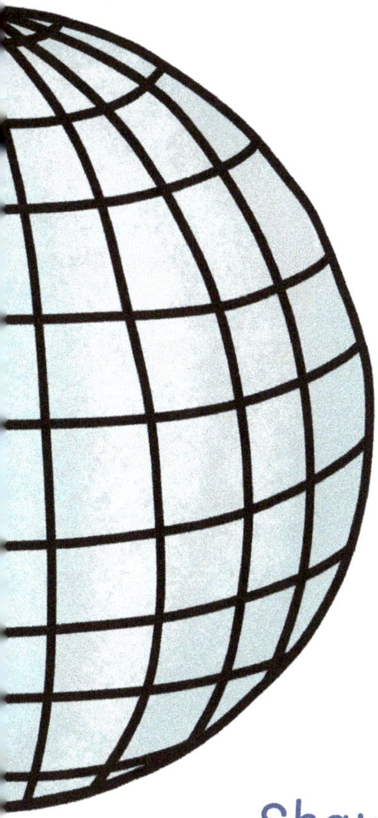

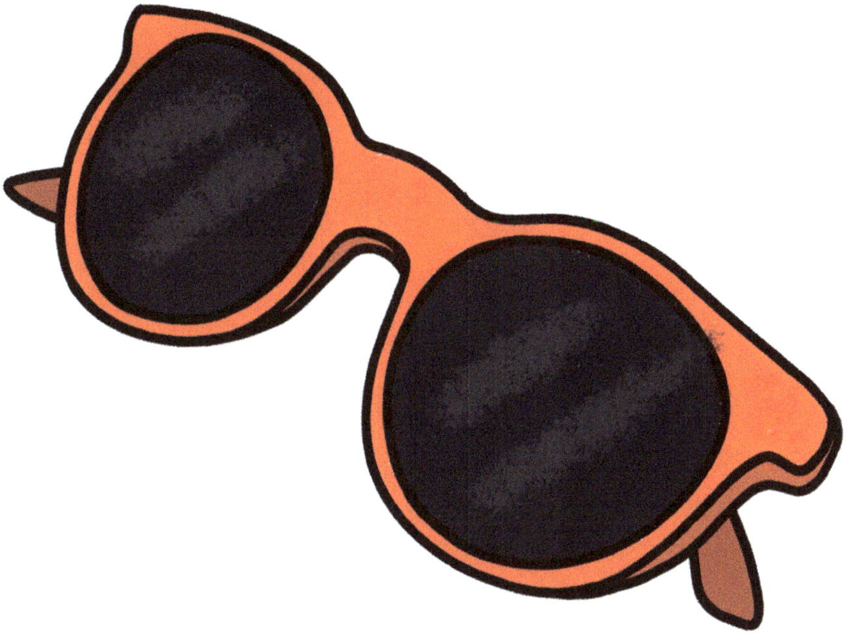

Shawn appreciates the artistic expression of music and how it inspires his creativity. Especially when it comes to his dance moves.

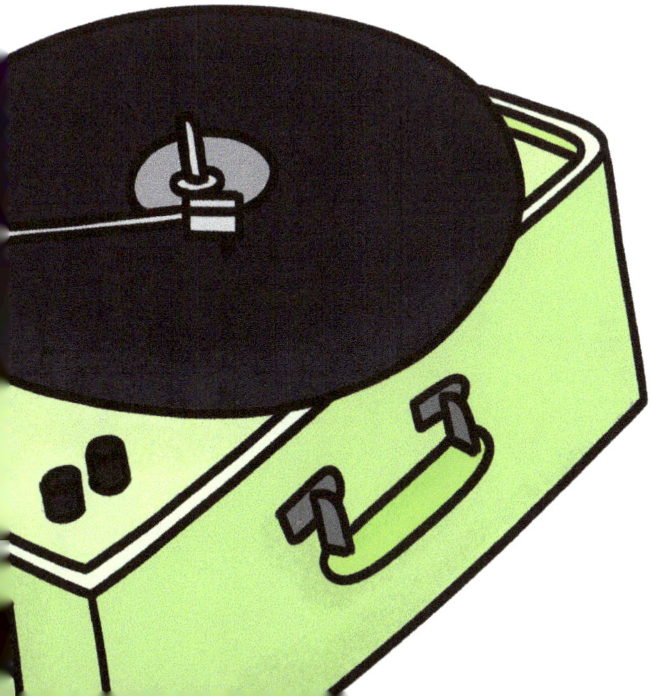

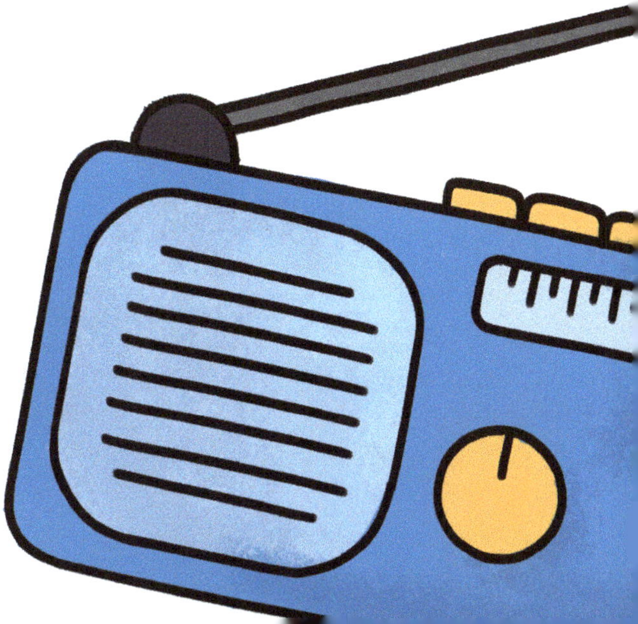

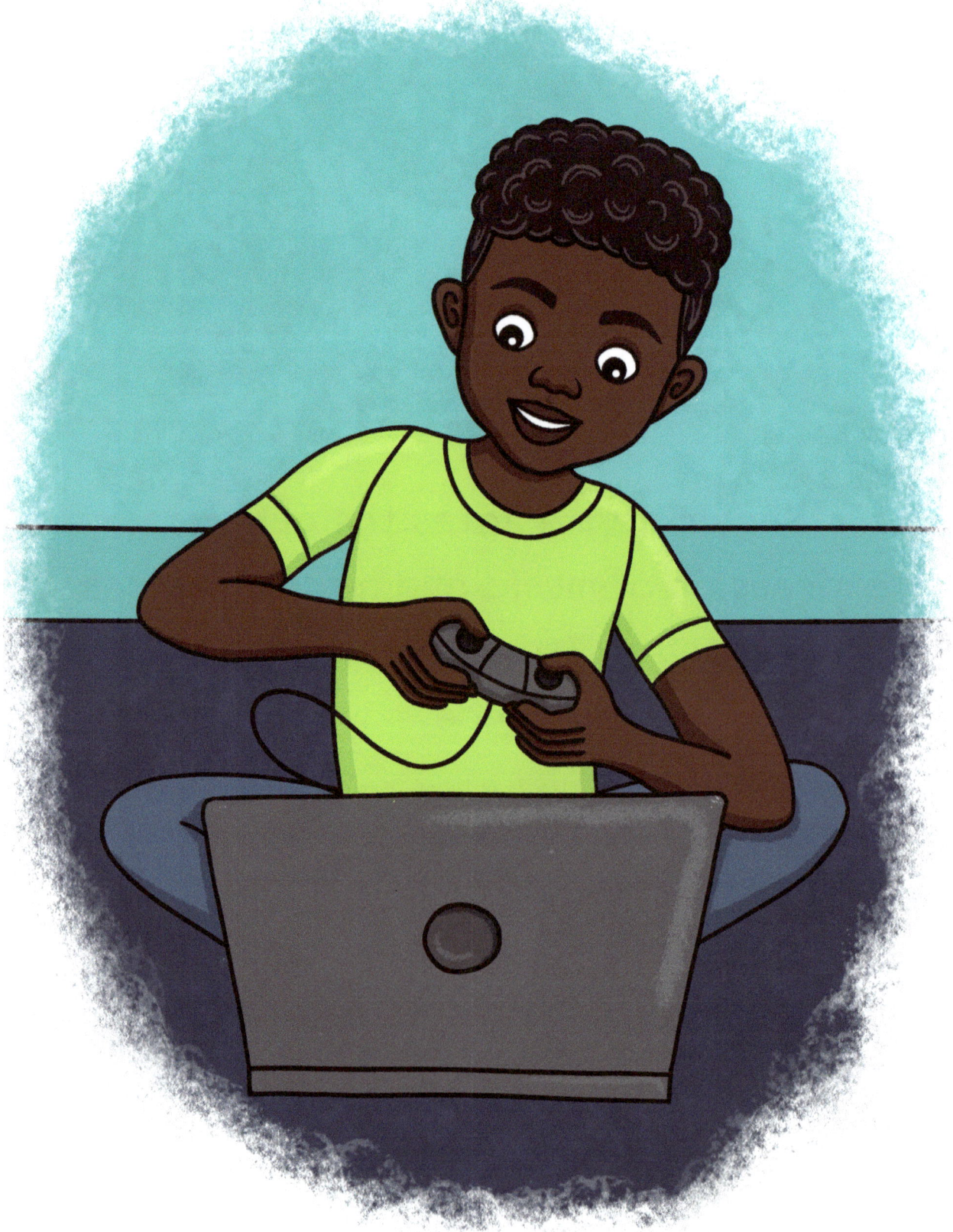

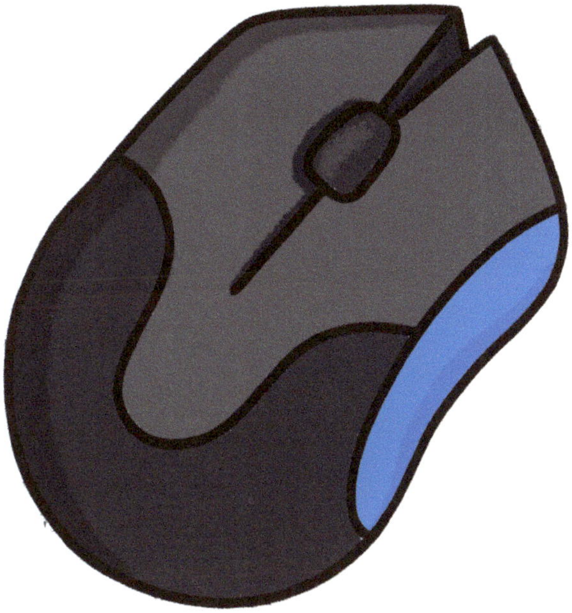

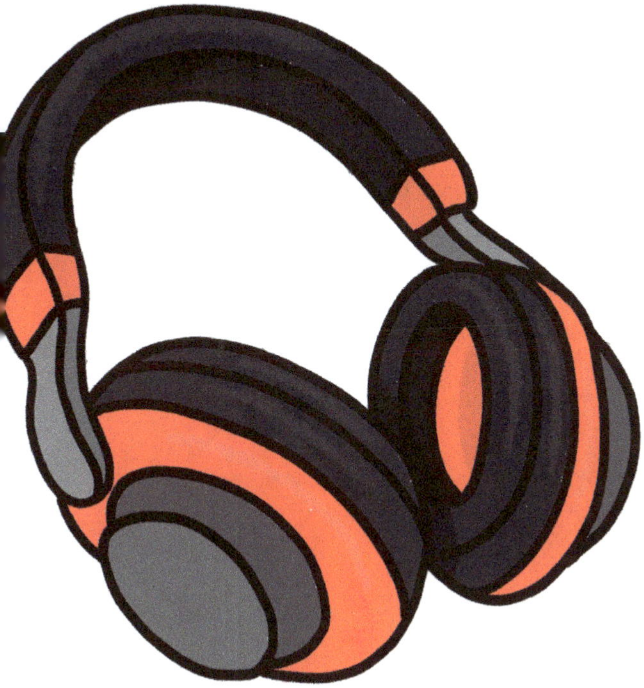

Shawn enjoys playing video games occasionally and traveling into the virtual world with his friends. As challenges present themselves, he joins forces with them to conquer the universe.

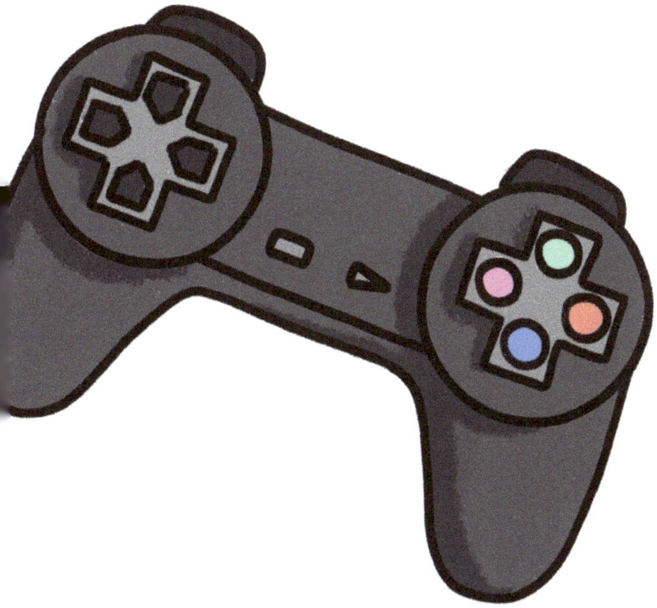

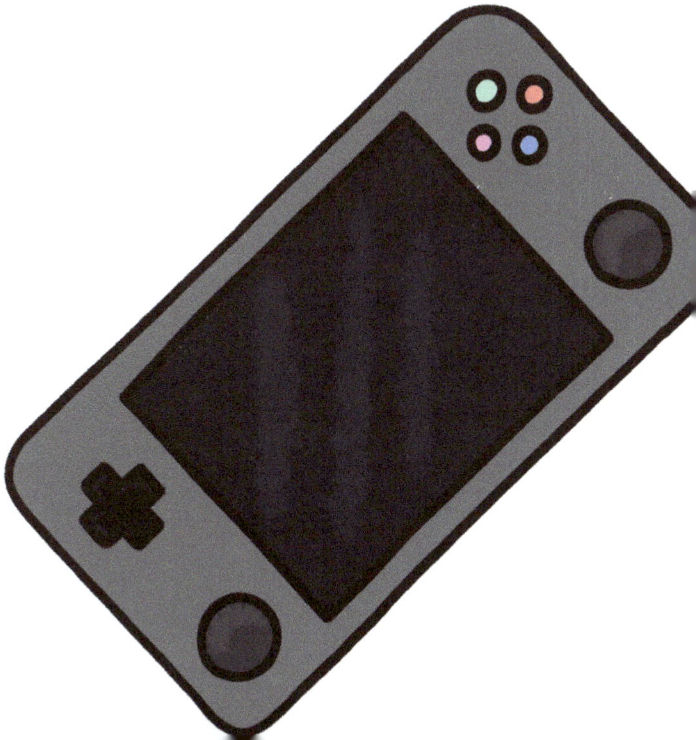

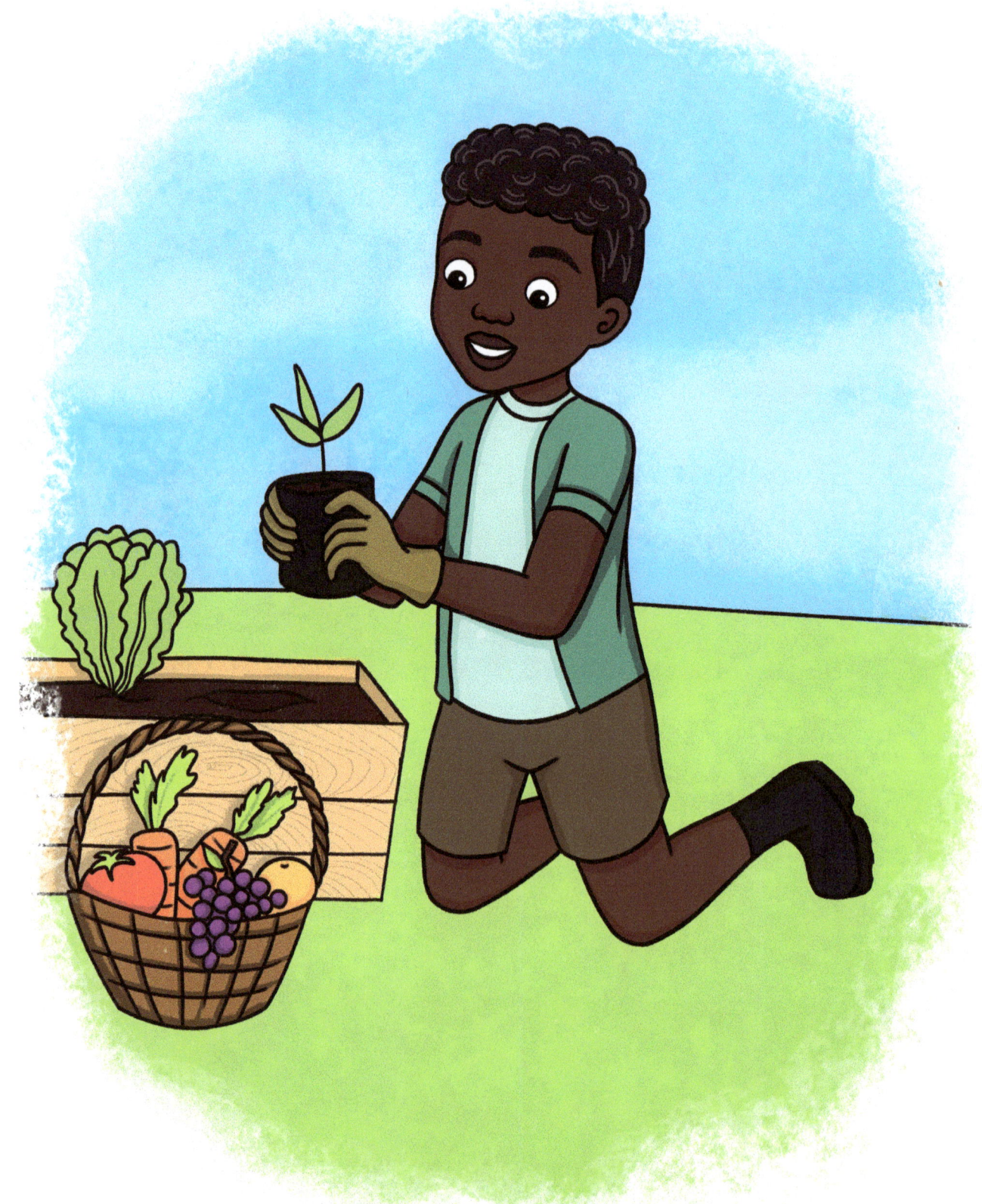

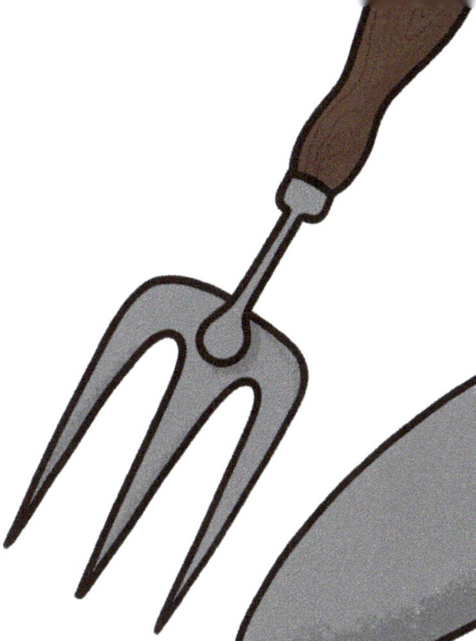

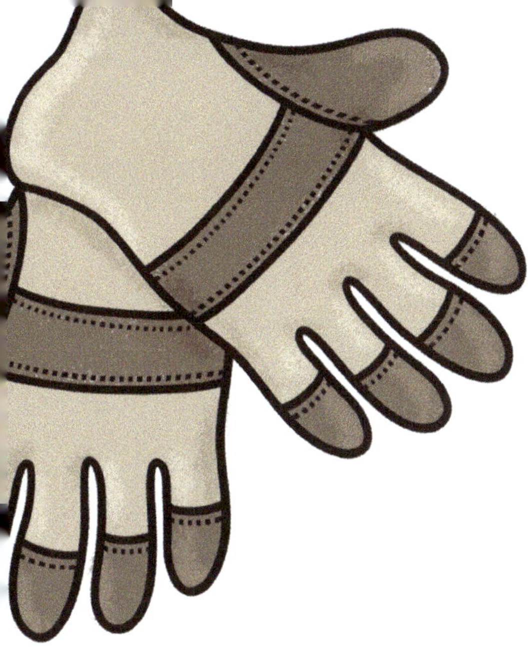

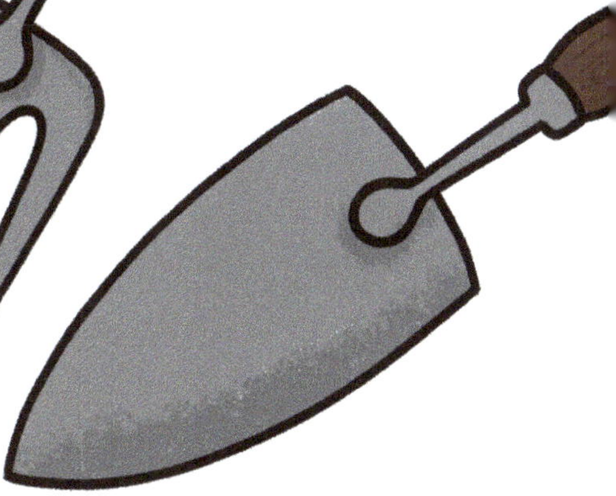

Shawn is fond of gardening for many reasons. His number one reason is how proud it makes him to grow the freshest, tastiest produce right in his back yard that he then gets to eat!

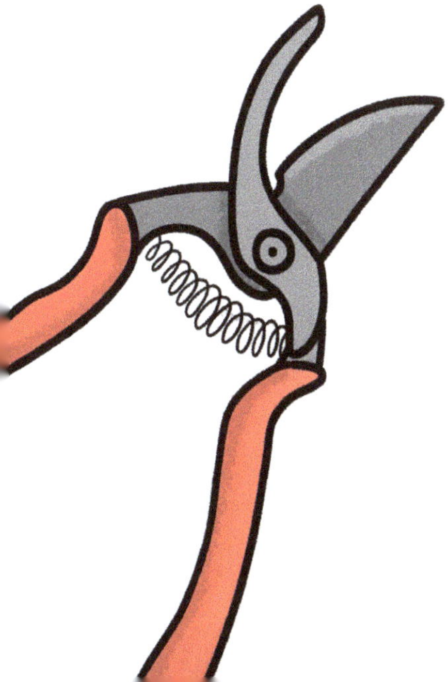

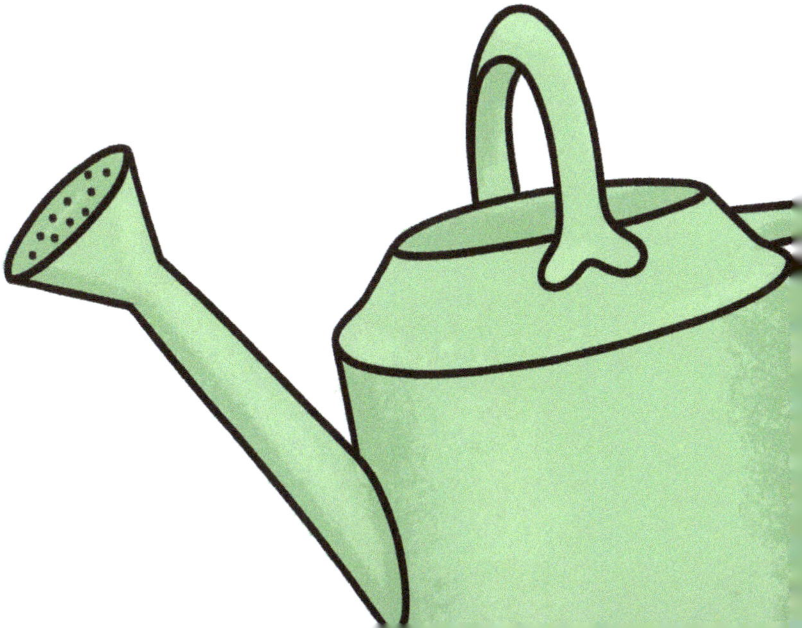

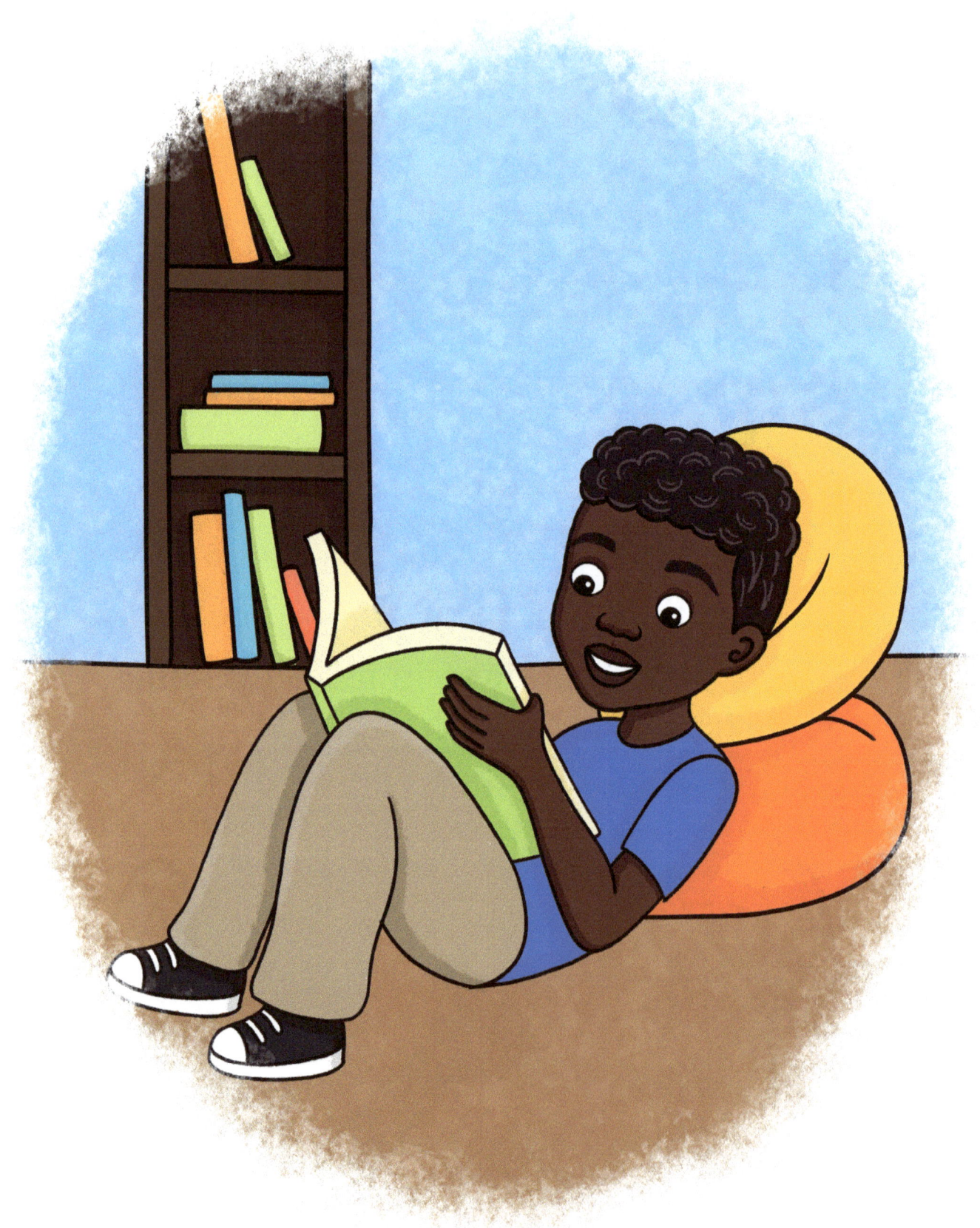

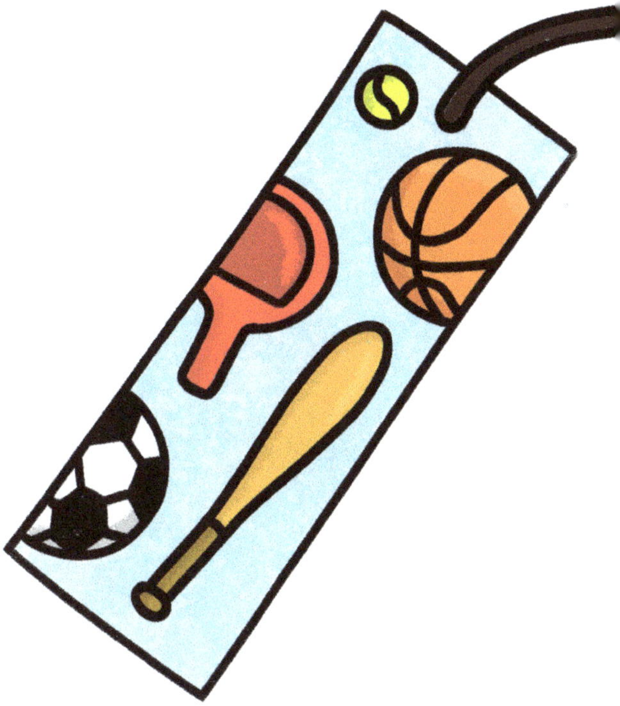

Reading has always been one of Shawn's favorite hobbies. Cuddling up with a good book keeps him laughing, learning, and a life-long fan of literature.

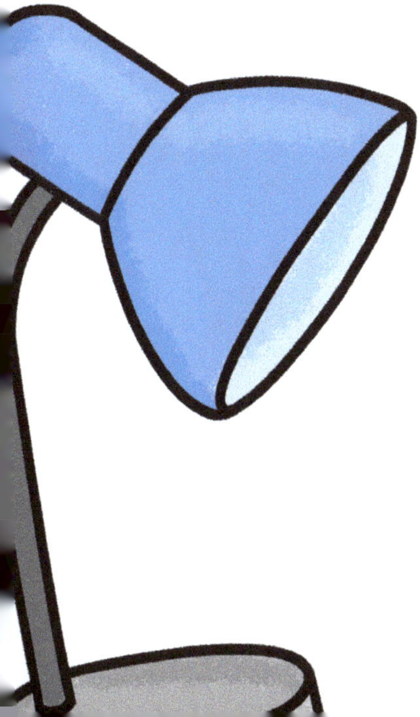

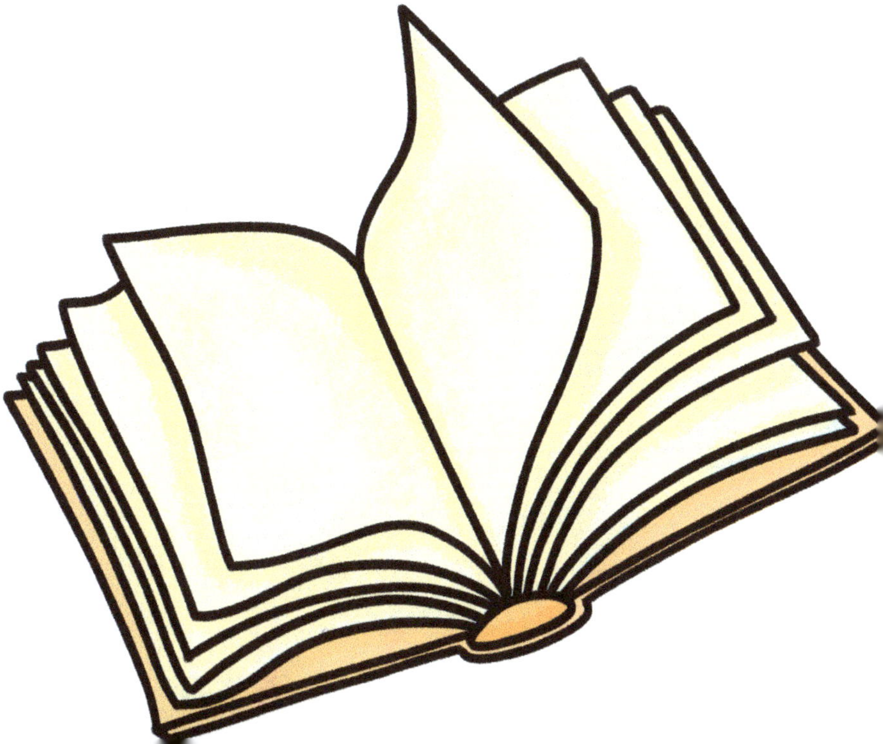

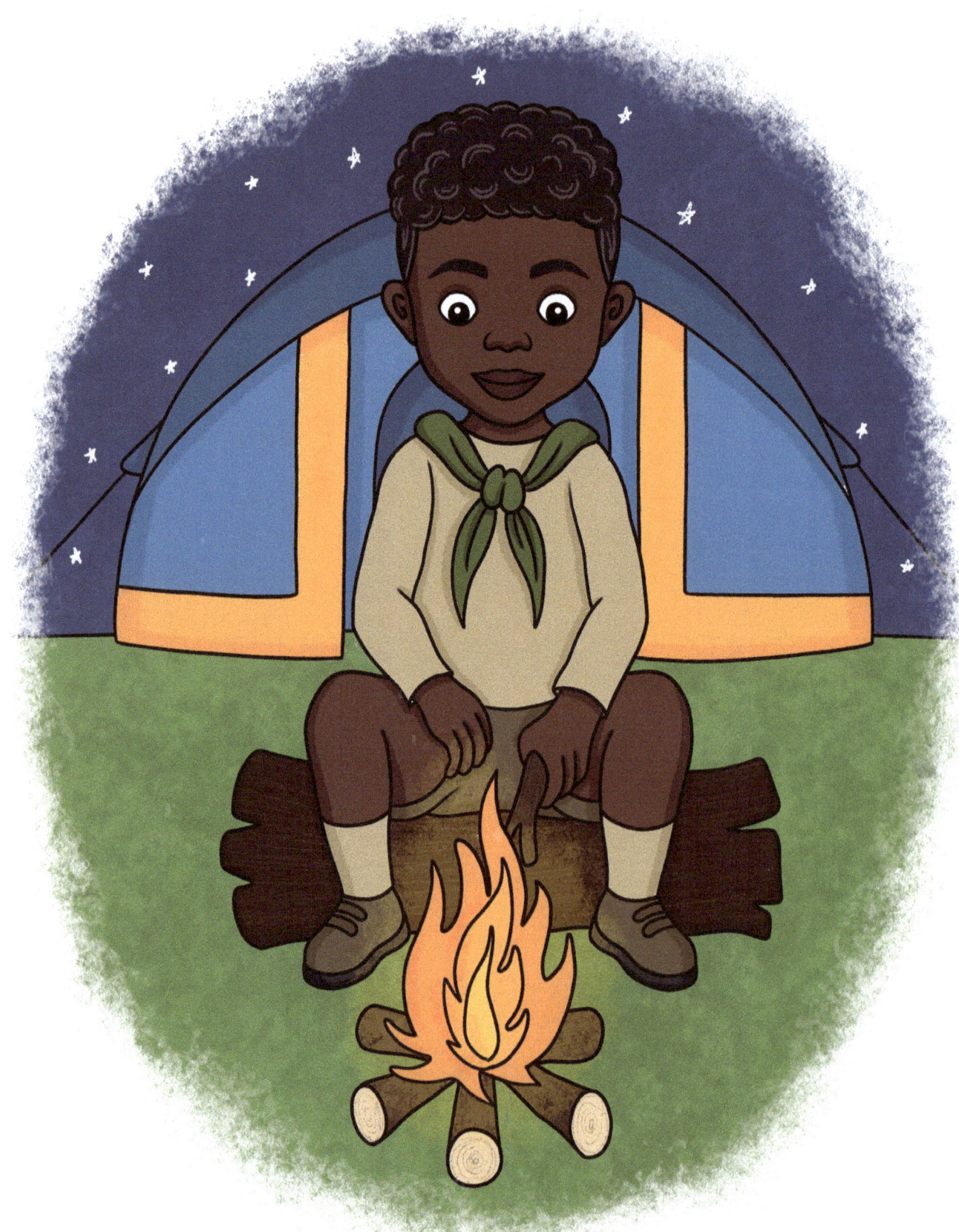

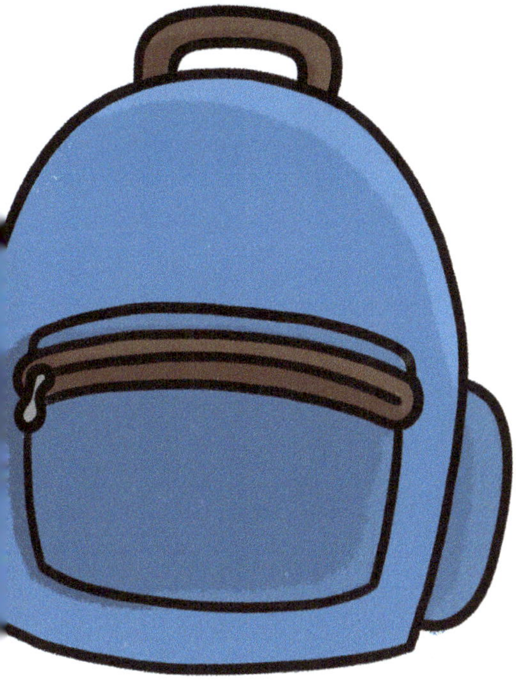

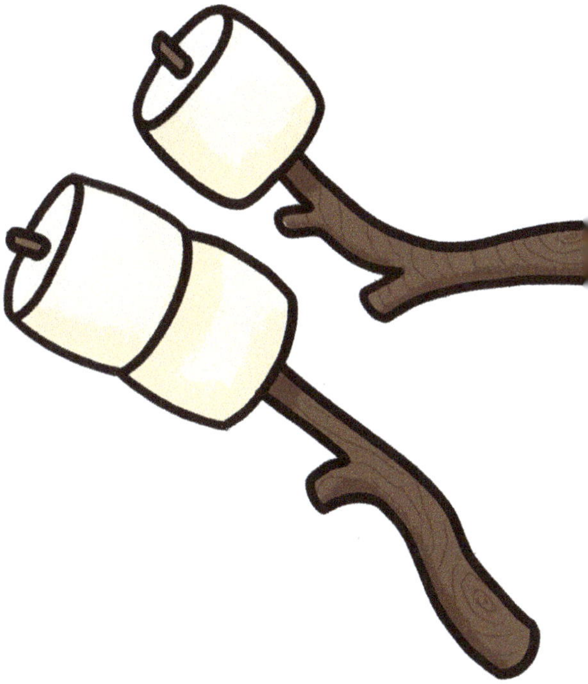

Camping helps Shawn unplug and become one with nature. The fresh air, campfire, and smores make for a great evening under the stars sharing entertaining stories.

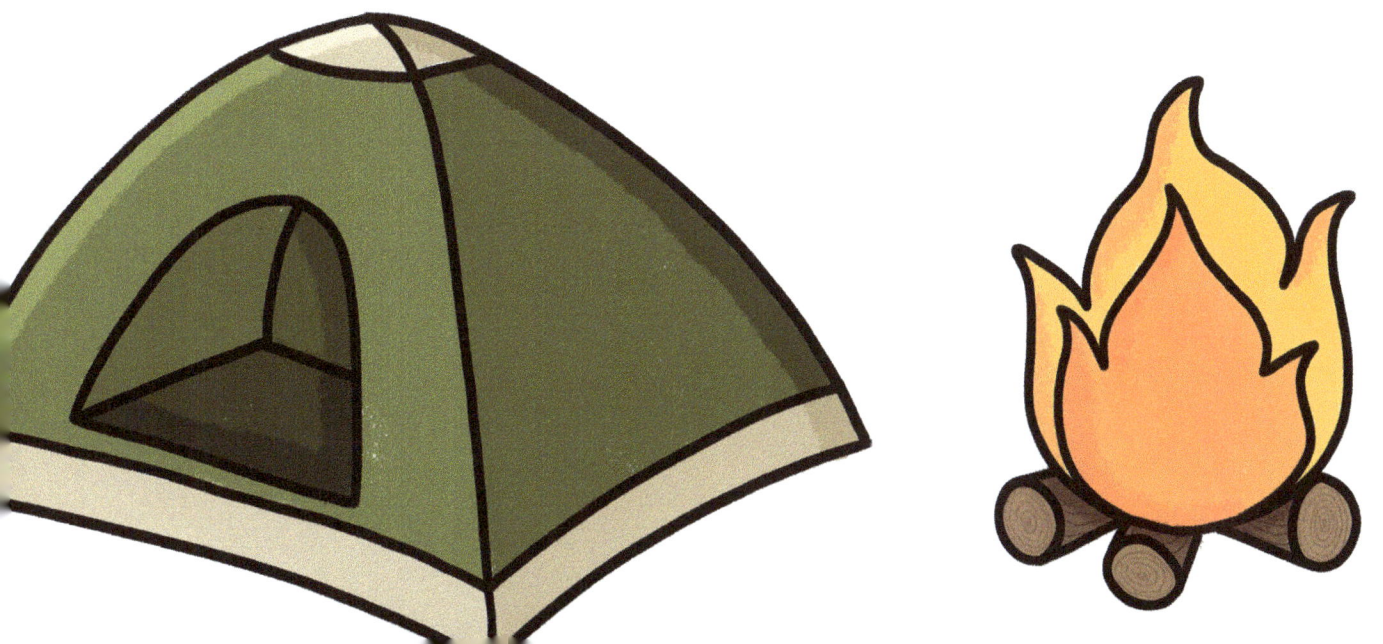

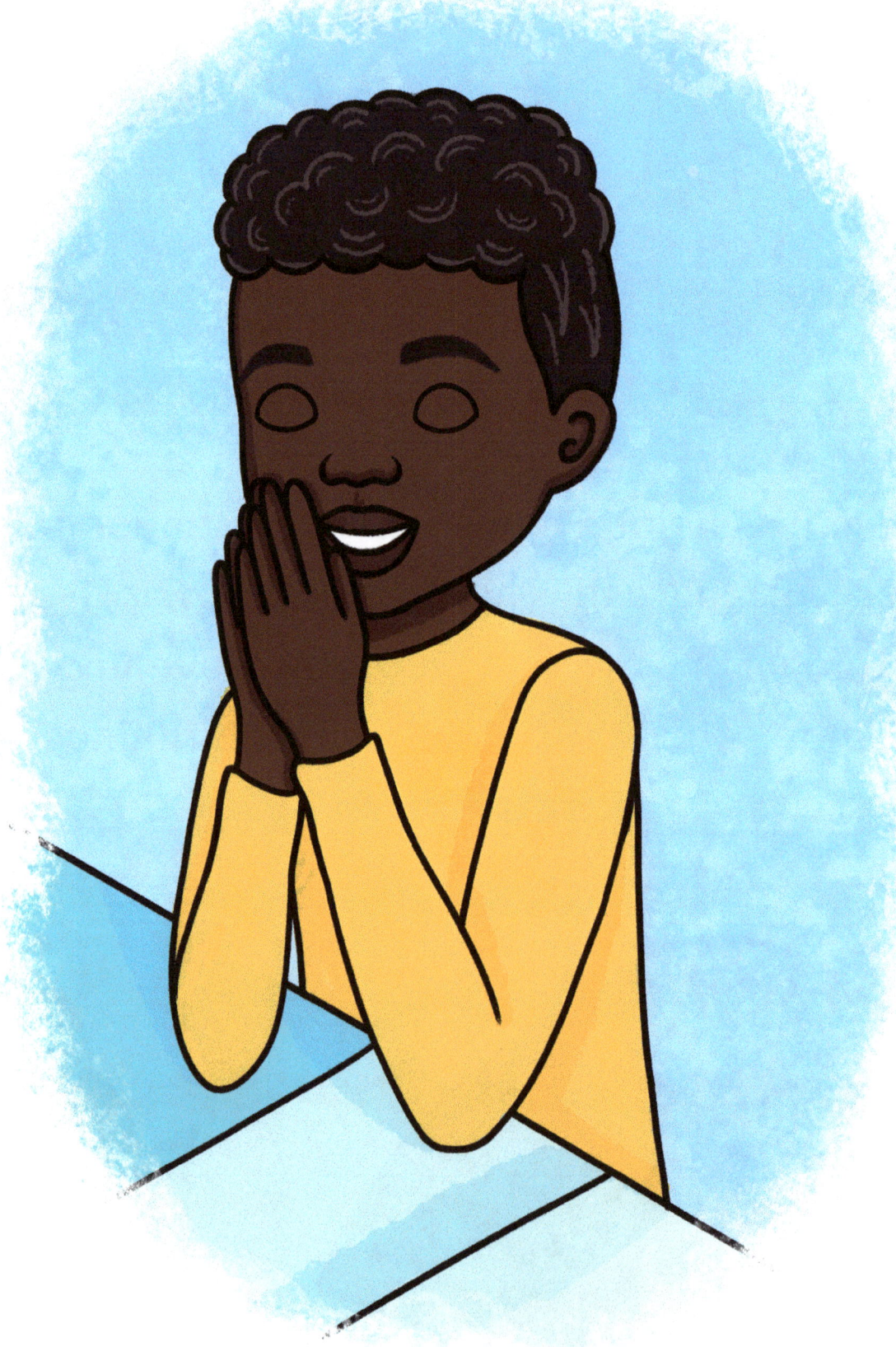

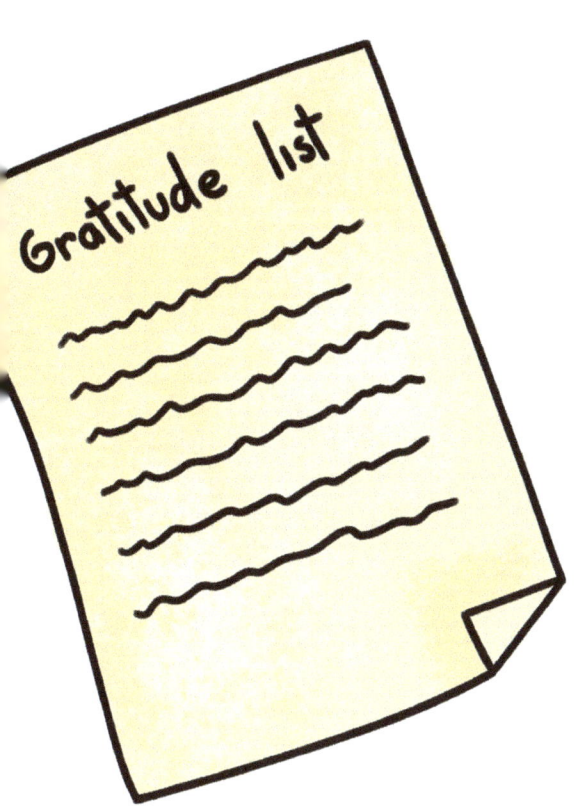
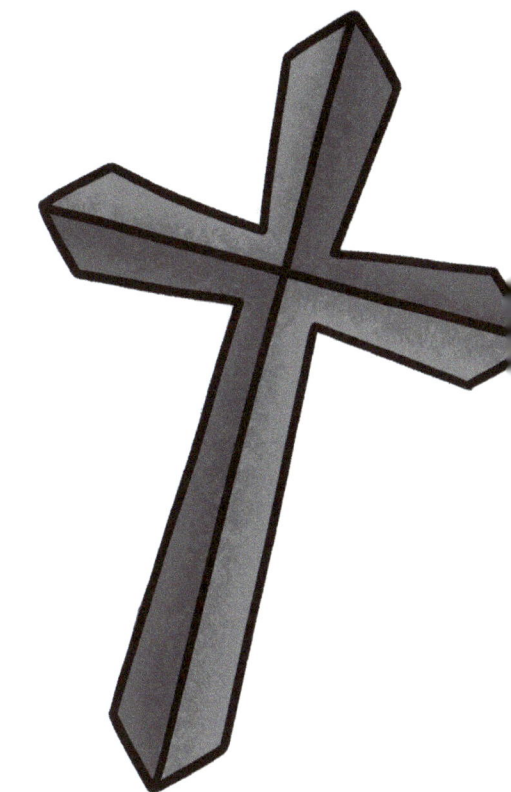

Shawn finds time every morning and evening to pray. He enjoys learning and reflecting on the word of God.

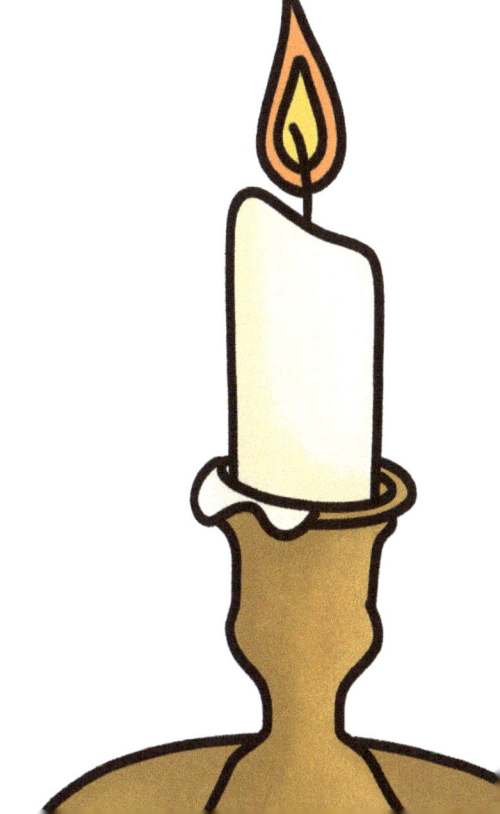

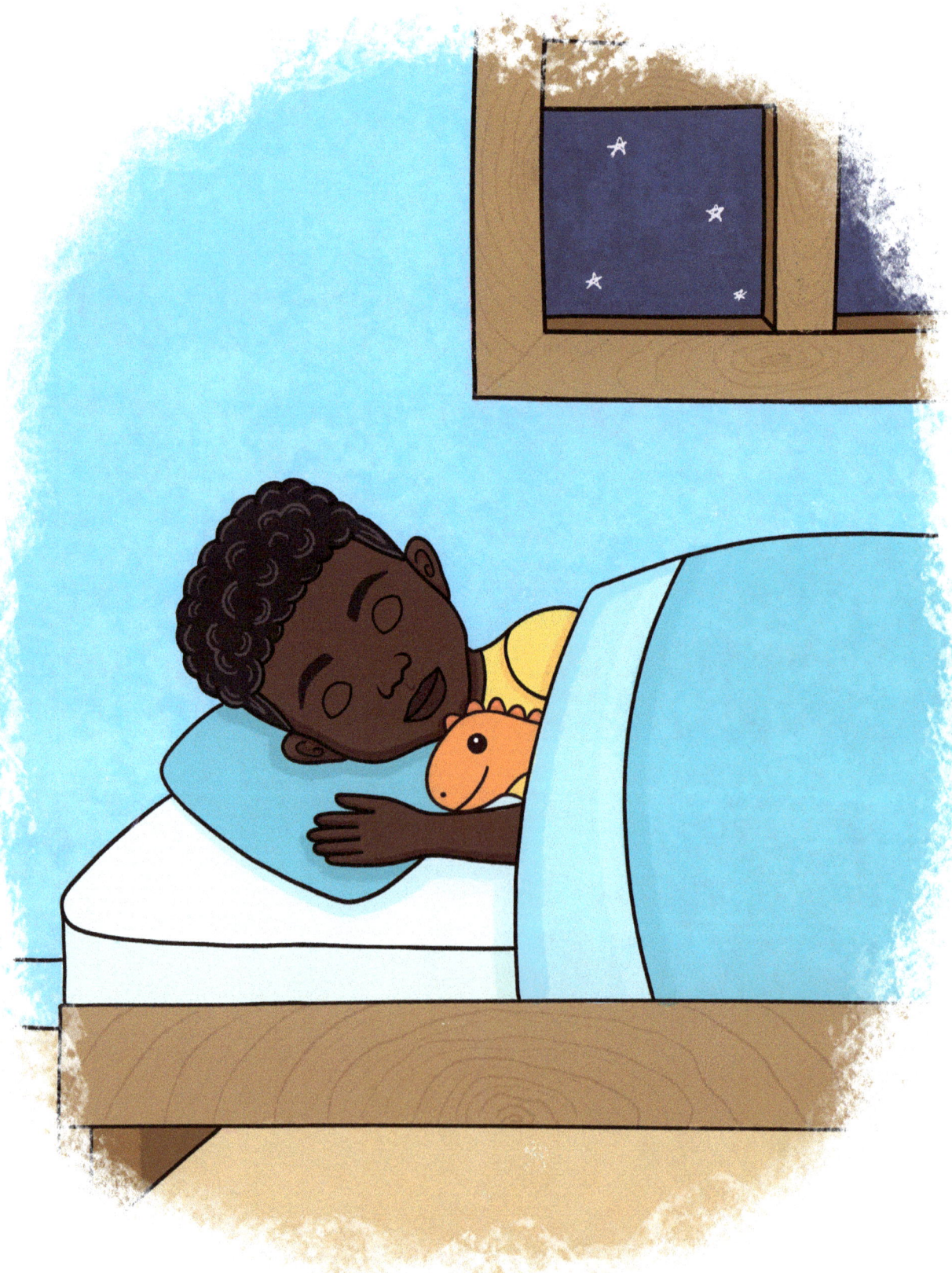

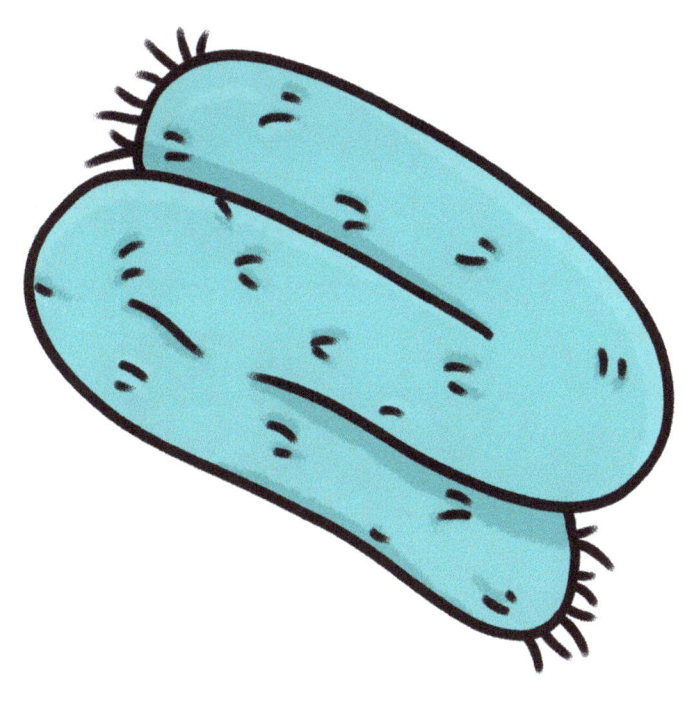

As much fun as Shawn has throughout the day, he knows the day must wind down. Sleep helps his body rest and recover for the adventures ahead.

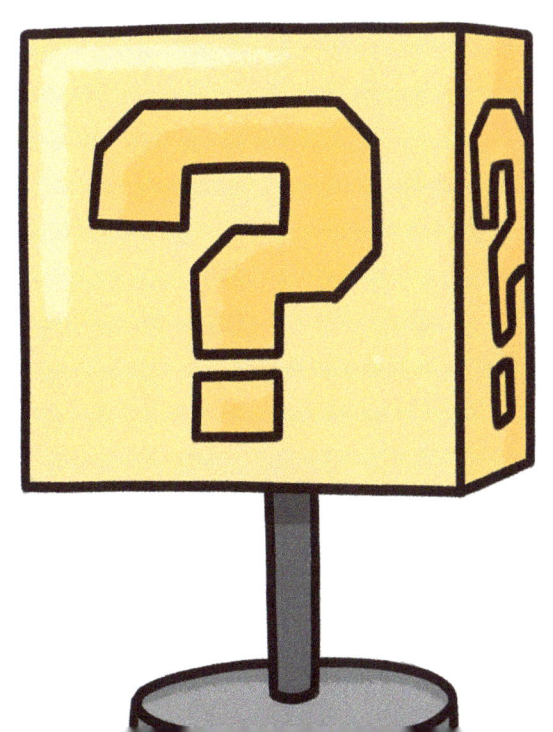
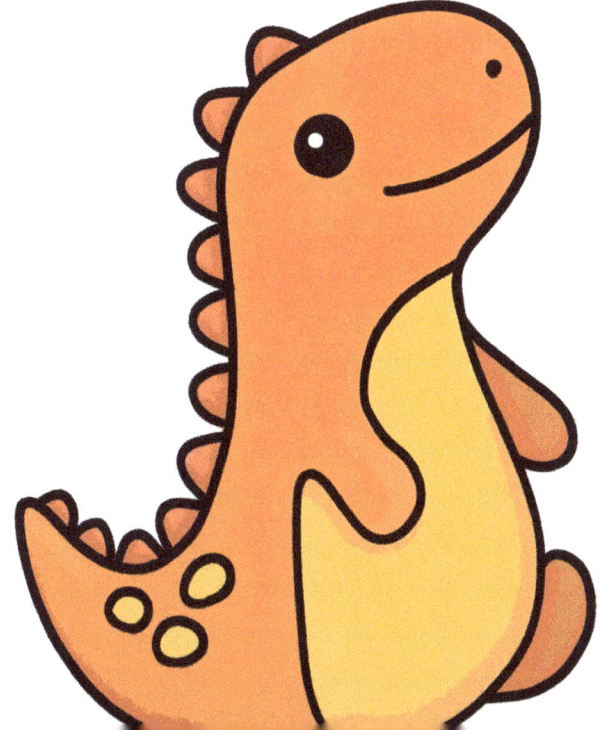

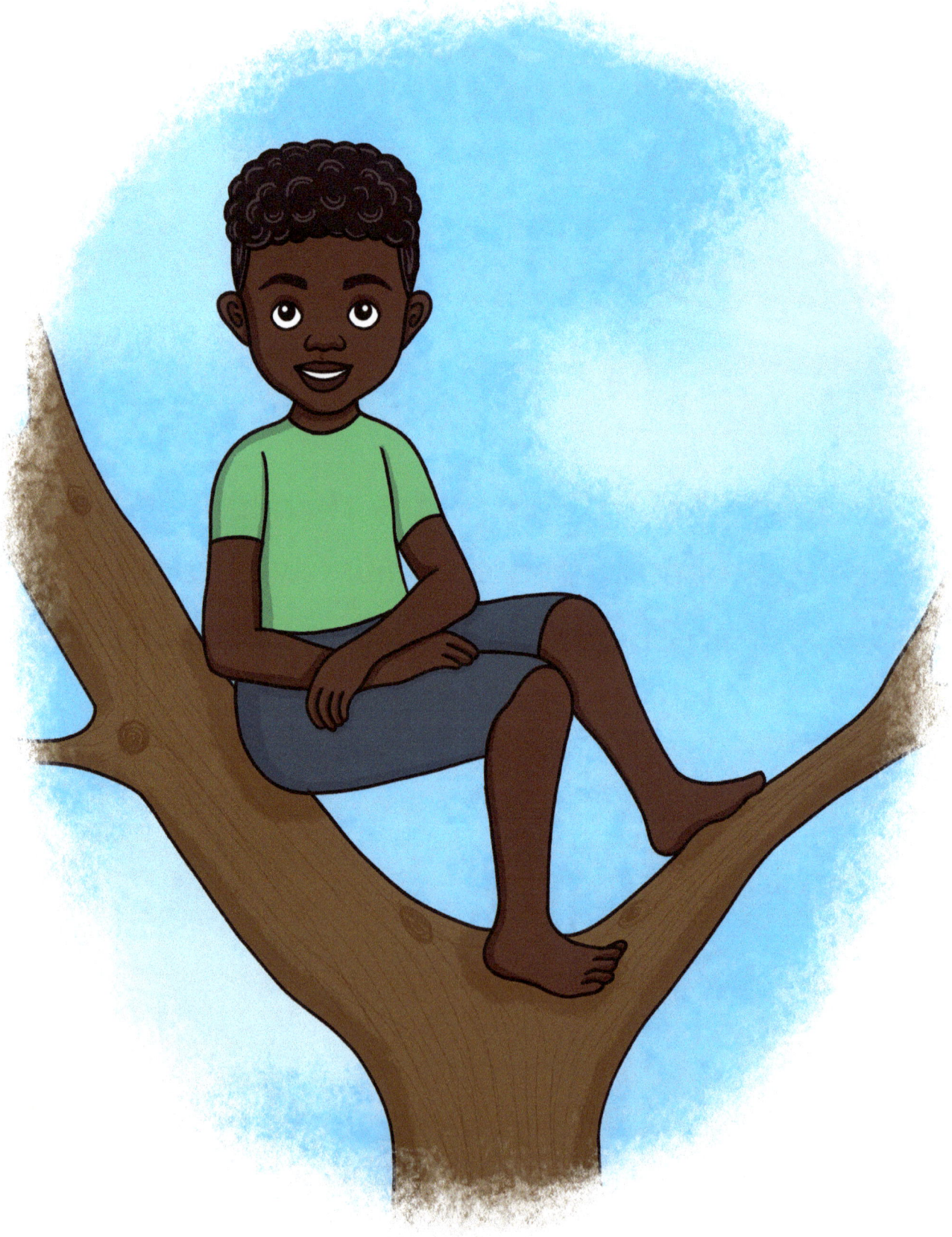

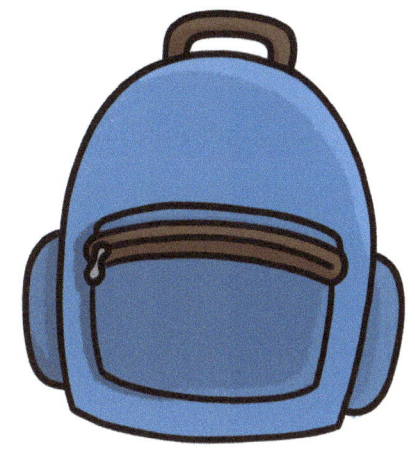
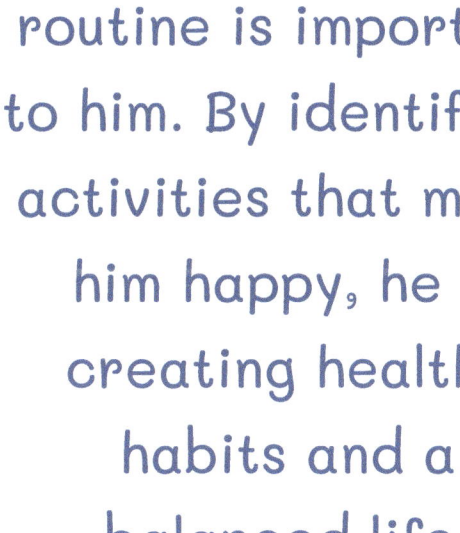
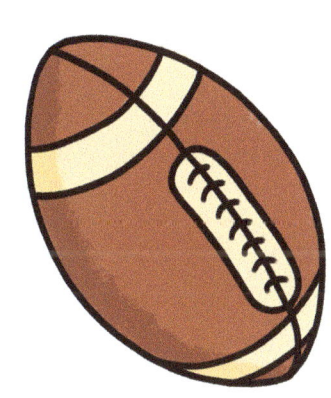

Shawn's self-care routine is important to him. By identifying activities that make him happy, he is creating healthy habits and a balanced life.

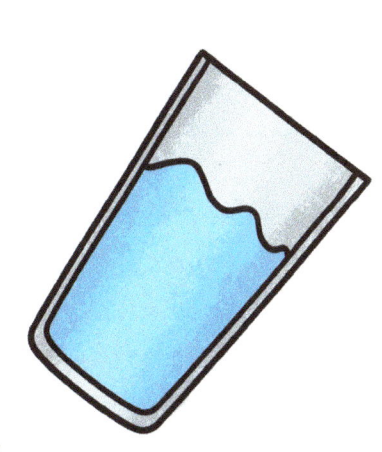
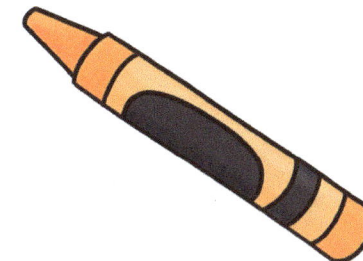
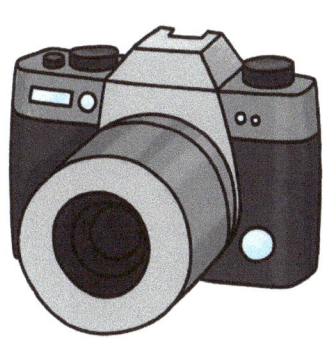

Self-Care is the best care. Take care of you and become the best version of your unique self. -DMJ

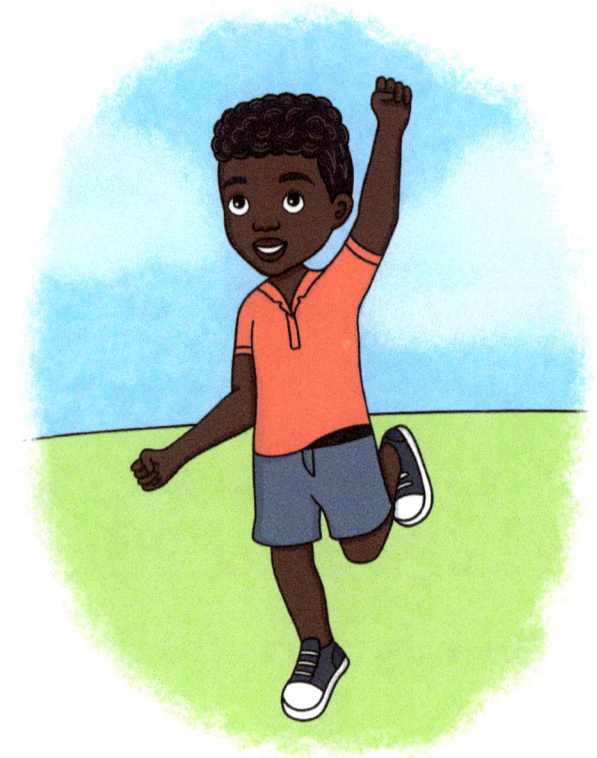

Shawn's Self-Care Routine:
A Boy's Guide to Healthy Habits
Copyright © 2022 by Hello Legendary Press LLC
Written by Danielle M. Jackson
Illustrated by Mariana Cadavid Suarez
ISBN 978-1-7361-5669-8
Library of Congress Control Number: 2022901491

All rights reserved. No part of this book may be used or reproduced in any manner whatsoever without the author's prior written permission. For information about permission to reproduce selections from this book and other work by the author, please visit www.hellolegendarypress.com/. Thank you for supporting the author's rights.

www.ingramcontent.com/pod-product-compliance
Lightning Source LLC
Chambersburg PA
CBHW051302110526
44589CB00025B/2917